Anna Dobbie

ENT Practice for Primary Care

D0309755

ENT Practice
for Primary Care

Andrew N. Coley MB ChB
General Practitioner and Hospital Practitioner in Otolaryngology
The Chestnuts Surgery, Poynton, Cheshire, UK

Nicholas J. Kay FRCSEng
Consultant ENT Surgeon
Stepping Hill Hospital, Cheshire, UK

SECOND EDITION
of ENT Practice for the GP's Surgery

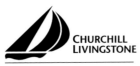

CHURCHILL
LIVINGSTONE

EDINBURGH LONDON MADRID MELBOURNE NEW YORK TOKYO 1998

CHURCHILL LIVINGSTONE
A Division of Harcourt Brace and Company Limited

© Harcourt Brace and Company 1998. All rights reserved.

 is a registered trademark of Harcourt Brace and Company Limited

No part of this publication may be reproduced, stored in a retrieval system,
or transmitted in any form or by any means, electronic, mechanical,
photocopying, recording or otherwise, without the prior permission of the
publishers (Harcourt Brace and Company Limited, 24–28 Oval Road, London
NW1 7DX), or a licence permitting restricted copying in the United Kingdom
issued by the Copyright Licensing Agency, 90 Tottenham Court Road,
London W1P 9HE.

ISBN 0–4430–6371–0

British Library Cataloguing in Publication Data
A catalogue record for this book is available from the British Library

Library of Congress Cataloging in Publication Data
A catalog record for this book is available from the Library of Congress

Medical knowledge is constantly changing. As new information becomes
available, changes in treatment, procedures, equipment and the use of drugs
becomes necessary. The authors and Publishers have, as far as it is possible,
taken care to ensure that the information given in the text is accurate and up
to date. However, readers are strongly advised to confirm that the
information, especially with regard to drug usage, complies with latest
legislation and standards of practice.

The Publishers and authors have made every effort to trace the copyright
holders for borrowed material. If they have inadvertently overlooked any,
they will be pleased to rectify the matter at the first opportunity.

The
Publisher's
policy is to use
paper manufactured
from sustainable forests

Commissioning Editor: Rachael Stock
Design direction: Ian Dick

Typeset by J&L Composition Ltd, Filey, North Yorkshire
Printed by Grafos S.A. Arte sobre papel, Spain

Preface to the second edition

It is 5 years since the first edition of this book which was well received by experienced practitioners and training registrars alike. This new edition has been created to reflect changes in the NHS, which have enabled specialised ENT practice to be undertaken within the general practice setting.

With the forthcoming development of Primary Care Groups there is a potential for great change in the strategic planning of the NHS and thus an alteration in the provision of care to patients. The suggestions in this book lay down some early ideas for critical care pathways over otolaryngogical problems and question where the provision of certain investigations and treatments are best placed. This is all part of a changing primary and secondary care interface.

It is with interest that the authors watch the change that comes with the 50th Anniversary of the NHS and reflect on the experience of service development here in the UK, and that found in the Health Maintenance Organisations of the USA.

The very helpful comments from general practitioners around the UK since the book was first published have been much appreciated and many are incorporated in this edition.

ANC   Stockport
NJK   1998

Preface

ENT problems, especially those in childhood, represent a high percentage of a GP's work load. Unfortunately, there is often little teaching in this subject; as a medical student, this amounts to one or two weeks during five years. Many doctors enter their trainee year with a large void in their knowledge of ENT problems.

Scanty teaching in otolaryngology has resulted in many general practitioners referring patients to hospital out-patient departments far sooner than they would prefer. A wider understanding of the history, examination and management of ENT problems may well result in GPs treating more of their patients within the surgery.

We have strenuously avoided the temptation of producing another comprehensive ENT textbook which, in general practice, would not really be useful. The topics cover the commonly presenting problems and their management in general practice and the text is, therefore, not a comprehensive account of specialist otolaryngology. Examination skills are only those used already and the equipment is no more than can be found in an average GP's surgery.

We feel that this book will be a useful addition to an individual practitioner's reference book collection. The format has been arranged to produce a 'user-friendly' guide, hopefully well-illustrated, to reduce the presence of text which takes time to read. It aims to offer a combination of easy reference and light reading when considering the common presenting ENT symptoms encountered in general practice. The chapters are arranged in such a way as to highlight areas quickly where:

- referral should be automatic
- management within the practice is appropriate and cost-effective
- useful management plans can be made for the middle ground between treatment and referral.

We hope this book will also become an asset in the general practice trainee year, encouraging useful discussion between trainer and trainee. For well-informed trainees to become competent and experienced principals, management of ENT problems will follow a sensible and well-thought out pattern.

This information may also encourage discussion between general practice principals and their local ENT consultants. This can only be beneficial and should improve patient care.

A.N.C.   Stockport
N.J.K.   1992

To our wives,
Ingrid and Barbara

Acknowledgements

We are indebted to Carolyn Saunders for invaluable skills and willingness in preparing the manuscript.

Our thanks are due to Dr John Sandars for his early encouragement and advice. Our thanks are due also to Abacus Studios (Stockport) for their photographic support.

A.N.C.   Stockport
N.J.K.   1998

Illustration acknowledgements
Figures: 2.4, 3.1A (5.3B), 3.1B (5.3E), 3.1C (5.3C), 3.1D (5.4), 3.2A, 3.2B, 3.4, 3.5, 3.6, 3.9, 4.1, 4.2, 4.4A (10.1B), 4.4B (10.1A), 4.5A, 4.5B, 5.3F. Hawke M et al 1990 Clinical Otoscopy: an introduction to ear diseases (2nd edn). Churchill Livingstone, Edinburgh.
Reproduced with permission of the authors and publishers.

Figures: 3.6 (4.3), 3.8, 10.2, 13.1, 13.5B, 14.1, 16.1, 21.1. Stafford ND and Youngs R 1988 Colour aids: ENT. Churchill Livingstone, Edinburgh.
Reproduced with permission of the authors and publishers.

Figures: 12.1, 16.2, 13.4, by courtesy of Prof N Stafford, Hull; 19.1, 19.2 by courtesy of Mr Alistair Gray FRCS, Stockport.

Contents

1

Equipment: basic requirements

The following equipment is recommended, most of which can be found in the GP's bag. Developments in the NHS now allow GPs to purchase materials and services which were originally confined to hospital practice. The basic equipment is considered below:

EARS

- *Otoscope*: it is most useful to have an otoscope with a swinging or sliding lens to facilitate combined inspection and instrumentation.

- *Tuning fork*: a 512 Hz fork (Fig. 1.1) with a sounding plate is the most desirable of the range; lower frequencies will be confused by the patient because of vibro-tactile sensation. A higher frequency will decay too quickly to enable Rinne's test to be effective.

- *Ear syringe*: the classic metal design is adequate (Fig. 1.2) but automatically pressured pumps (Fig. 1.3) are also relatively

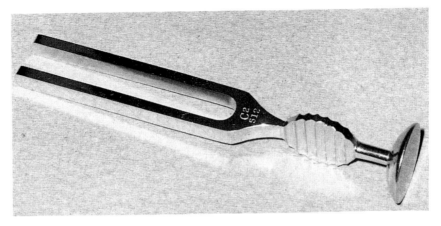

Fig. 1.1 A 512 Hz tuning fork.

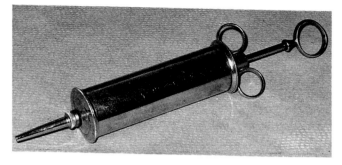

Fig. 1.2 Classic metal design ear syringe.

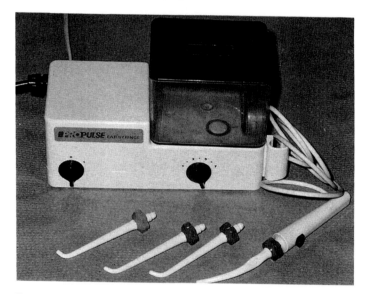

Fig. 1.3 Modern automatically pressured pump for ear syringing.

inexpensive and well worth considering to remove meatal wax.

- *Picture discrimination cards*: the authors use the Leeds Picture Discrimination Cards which are phoneme-matched pictures (Fig. 1.4).

NOSE

- An *otoscope* can be used with a large speculum. The patient should not breathe through the nose during this brief examination or else the lens will steam up.

- *A cosmetic mirror* will show nasal patency by virtue of steaming up when held under the nose; this is especially useful in assessing very young children and babies.

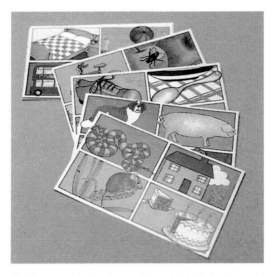

Fig. 1.4 Leeds Picture Discrimination Cards designed by Dr Mabel Yates.

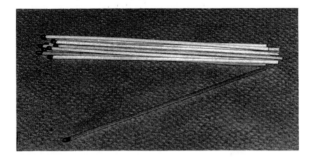

Fig. 1.5 Silver nitrate cautery sticks.

- *Silver nitrate sticks* (Fig. 1.5) are useful in dealing with septal varicose vessels that are causing epistaxes. This is a straight-forward procedure which is covered in Chapter 14.

THROAT

- *Wooden tongue depressors* are abundant in the surgery.

- A *powerful pencil torch* is recommended for examination of the oral cavity and oropharynx.

- *Disposable gloves* will be needed for palpation of the floor of the mouth and buccal sulci.

Those colleagues who have had formal ENT training will be adept at using a head mirror and incident light to free both hands for instrumentation. An office desk lamp with a 100 watt bulb will suffice.

Primary Care Groups and Health Authorities can now purchase additional more specialised services to offer more direct health care for the patient.

The local GP is well placed to understand the needs of the local populus and can liaise with the willing providers, e.g. audiology services within the practice. Fund-holding experience has shown that this is a cost-effective service and allows the development of the primary and secondary care interface. This is apparent in the case of audiometry and tympanometry which enables the GP to make a more informed referral thus facilitating the specialist consultation.

These developing ideas will be discussed in each chapter where appropriate and may well serve as a starting point for critical care pathways.

2

Equipment: application

An ENT examination requires good technique which is easy in the cooperative adult but not in a baby or anxious young child. Assistance will be needed from either a sensible parent or sympathetic member of staff in the surgery; this is portrayed in Figures 2.1 and 2.2, without labouring the point any further in text. Further elaboration and illustration can be found in the appropriate chapters.

EARS

Key points:
- Presence of scars (Fig. 2.3)
- Deformity of pinna
- Appearance of external auditory canals
- Appearance of tympanic membranes (Fig .2.4)

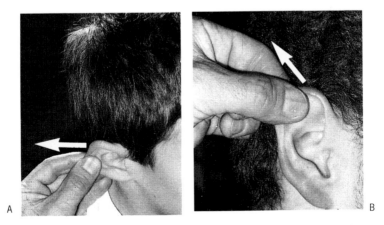

A   B

Fig. 2.1 A A child's ear should be retracted gently posteriorly prior to inserting the auriscope. **B** An adults' ear should be retracted posterosuperiorly prior to inserting the auriscope.

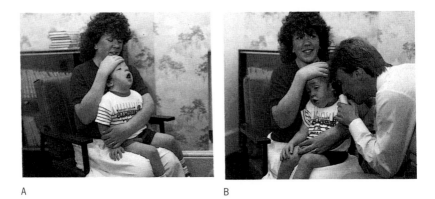

Fig. 2.2 Suggested techniques for examining the mouth and ears in a young child.

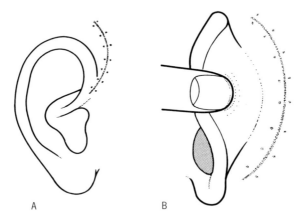

Fig. 2.3 A Scar of an endaural incision. **B** Scar of a postaural incision, seen by retracting the pinna forward.

NOSE

Key points:
- Linearity
- Patency of each nostril (Fig. 2.5)
- Little's area; i.e. that area of the septum visible on tilting the nasal tip upwards
- Vestibules
- Septum
- Turbinates (inferior turbinates are the most visible)

MOUTH, THROAT AND NECK

Key points:
- Scars or swellings
- Facial and lip symmetry

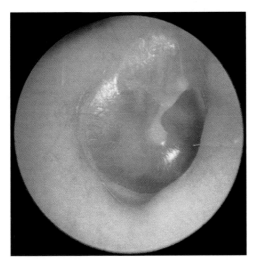

Fig. 2.4 Normal tympanic membrane.

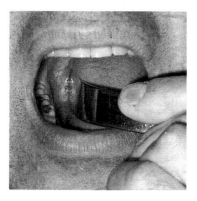

Fig. 2.5 Misting of a mirror confirms nasal patency in a young child.

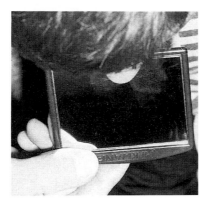

Fig. 2.6 Retromolar trigone shown by tongue retraction.

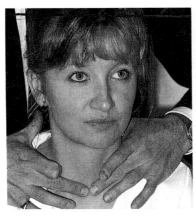

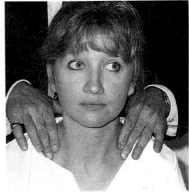

Fig. 2.7 A Start with the suprasternal notch.

Fig. 2.7 B Move laterally to supraclavicular fossae.

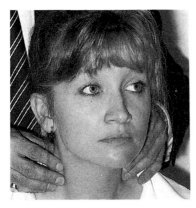

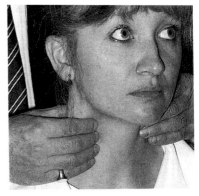

Fig. 2.7 C Check the posterior triangles.

Fig. 2.7 D Remember to palpate around the sternomastoid muscles.

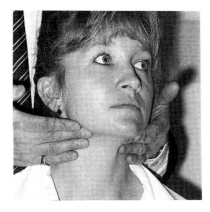

Fig. 2.7 E Finish off with submandibular areas.

- Quality of speech
- Teeth
- Hard palate
- Tongue appearance and movement
- Buccal mucosa including retromolar trigone (Fig. 2.6)
- Palpation of floor of mouth and buccal sulci; palpation of neck; this should be done in an orderly manner (Figs 2.7 A–E)

3

Earache

- Earache is a common presenting symptom in general practice; it is often indicative of an ear infection although, if the ears are both normal, a referred cause should be sought.

- Glue ear may cause an acute otitis media or vice versa.

- Rigid classification of presenting problems and differential diagnosis is difficult but the following tabulation is suggested as a useful guide based on the clinical experience of the authors.

- The possible findings in cases of suspected ear infection are listed below but these must be considered in conjunction with the history.

POINTS OF HISTORY

Viral otitis media	Bacterial otitis media
Secondary to URTI or exanthemata	May follow viral otitis media
Recent onset (<36 h)	May be a complication of tonsillitis
Mild pyrexia	Marked pyrexia
	More often unilateral
May present in conjunction with diarrhoea and vomiting in younger children	Infrequent vomiting may be a secondary feature
Discharge of liquid wax	Purulent and bloody discharge from a spontaneous perforation associated with pain relief

Overall deafness if both ears are affected

FINDINGS ON OTOSCOPY

Viral otitis media	Bacterial otitis media
Handle of malleus flush (Fig. 3.1A)	Red and bulging (Fig. 3.1D)
Bubbles sometimes seen behind membrane in conjunction with above findings (Fig. 3.1B)	Haemorrhagic areas on membrane
Dull tympanic membrane, i.e. diminished or no light reflex (Fig. 3.1C)	Central perforation associated with pulsatile discharge of pus
Peripheral vessels (Fig. 3.1E)	

NB Causative features, e.g. coryza, tonsillitis, should be sought.

MANAGEMENT OF EARACHE

Initial presentation is within a few hours of onset of earache; this is often reported during out-of-hours emergency cover.

● Instruct on the use of paracetamol for the next 12–24 hours because pain is the most severe symptom. The rationale for witholding antibiotics at this stage is that immunoglobulins within the exudate in the middle ear may well cope alone with the infection. This witholding of antibiotics at this early stage must be explained to the parents in order to prevent any breakdown of their confidence.

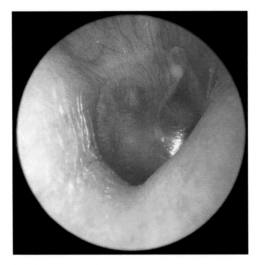

Fig. 3.1 A Malleus flush.

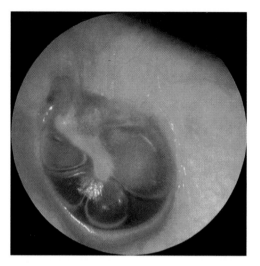

Fig. 3.1 B Bubbles behind the tympanic membrane in this ear were due to otitic barotrauma, but similar findings can also be seen in secretory otitis media.

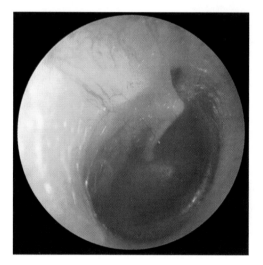

Fig. 3.1 C Dull tympanic membrane.

- Ensure that the parent understands the rationale that viral otitis media is often self-limiting and that antibiotics are not immediately necessary.

- If earache persists for more than 24 hours, further GP review is necessary to treat a likely bacterial otitis media with appropriate antibiotics but do consider the possibility of ampicillin-resistant haemophilus and streptococci.

- The GP may find it necessary to review the child in two weeks to exclude secretory otitis media (syn. glue ear, Fig. 3.2) as this

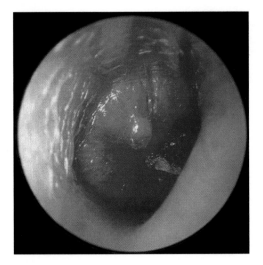

Fig. 3.1 D Bulging tympanic membrane.

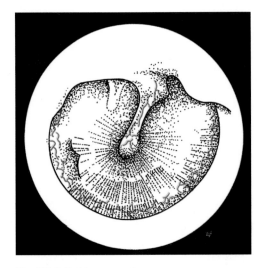

Fig. 3.1 E Peripheral vessels.

may explain a previous history of recurrent earache; the vicious cycle of glue ear and recurrent acute otitis media should always be borne in mind.

- Secretory otitis media has to be bilateral if there is free-field deafness (see Ch. 5).

- Recurrent acute otitis media causing parental or GP concern:
  REFER

- For the child with recurrent low-grade earache, a prolonged course of low dose antibiotic, e.g. trimethoprim (2 mg per kg at

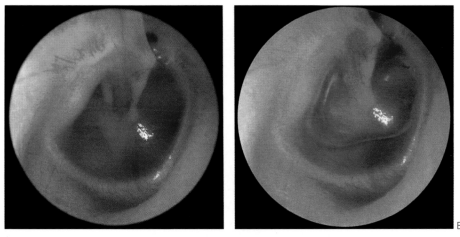

Fig. 3.2 Secretory otitis media **A** Honey-coloured tympanic membrane. **B** Air-fluid meniscus.

night), for 8 weeks may allow the situation to resolve without the need for referral.

- Persistent earache complicated by ear discharge: **REFER**
- Earache with history of underlying ear disease needs investigation: **REFER**
- If tympanic membrane looks normal, see 'Other Local Causes'.

Sequelae of viral and bacterial otitis media

- Complete resolution: no further action
- Recurrence of earache: see above
- Secretory otitis media
  - asymptomatic: observe
  - deafness (see Ch. 5)
  - leading onto recurrent otitis media: consider using low dose trimethoprim as outlined previously
  - acute otitis media de novo is less common in adults than in childhood and a history of previous ear disease should be sought

The role of the specialist team

- Most referrals for recurrent earache occur in children with glue ear.
- Parents should be reassured that glue ear is age-related (Fig. 3.3) and the role of management is to **palliate** until natural resolution occurs.
- The specialist will likely build on the conservative management as outlined above.

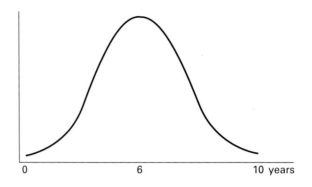

Fig. 3.3 Age v incidence of secretory otitis media.

- Grommets are used to ventilate the middle ear and are effective in the palliation of symptoms but are only used when non-surgical management has failed.

- Some situations may require repeated grommet insertion +/- adenoidectomy; the role of adenoidectomy as a specific contribution will vary according to the local specialist opinion.

- Acute perforation (Fig. 3.4) may heal spontaneously. Advise against water and shampoos entering the ear. Observe and review in one month to ensure complete resolution.

- Chalk patches (syn. tympanosclerosis) (Fig. 3.5) is a long-term sequel to infection: no action.

- Chronic perforations (see Ch. 10).

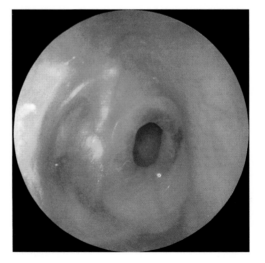

Fig. 3.4 Acute otitis media resulting in a temporary perforation.

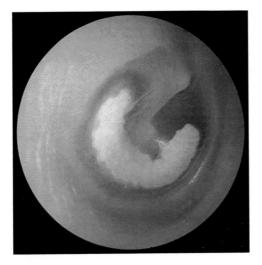

Fig. 3.5 Tympanosclerosis.

OTHER LOCAL CAUSES

Otitis externa

Primary otitis externa represents eczema and secondary infection of skin in the external auditory canal and meatal orifice, sometimes involving the pinna. It is usually (but not always) bilateral and includes the following features:

- Itch or ache
- Discharge, usually watery
- Slight deafness or fullness
- Aching down the neck from associated external jugular glands

Management

- If very mild with minimal debris, use trial of antibiotic/steroid mixture drops, three times a day for 5 days e.g. gentamicin and hydrocortisone compound. Avoid shampoo and bath water contamination by using cotton wool pledgets smeared with petroleum jelly.

- If a primary care nurse is ENT trained, then a broad spectrum antibiotic cream on $\frac{1}{2}$ inch ribbon gauze can be introduced, three times a week (Fig. 3.6); if not **REFER** .

- If condition fails to settle **REFER** for microsuction (see Ch. 4)

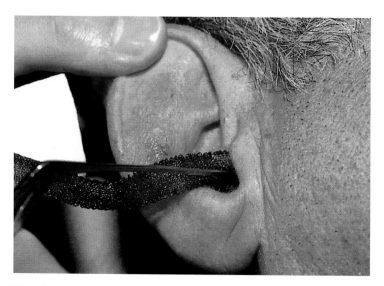

Fig. 3.6 Ear packed with ½-inch ribbon gauze. The above example shows a glycerine and ichthammol wick, but where there is a reasonably wide lumen, an antibiotic cream can be used.

PITFALLS

Unilateral otitis externa may be:

- Traumatic in origin

- Secondary to a perforation. If perforation is suspected by pulsatile debris/discharge **REFER** for microsuction and examination

- Pseudomonal otitis externa

Furuncle

- A staphylococcal boil in external auditory meatus of one ear (Fig. 3.7)

- Very painful

- Diagnosed by pulling upwards and backwards; the pain is made worse during this manoeuvre

Treatment

- Glycerin and ichthammol on ½ inch ribbon gauze (see Fig. 3.6)

- Analgesics by mouth although if patient is debilitated by pain and loss of sleep, **REFER** urgently for in-patient management

- Seven days of the appropriate dose of flucloxacillin

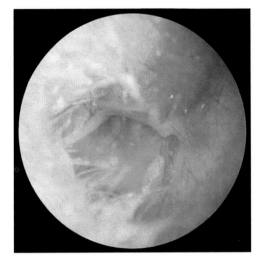

Fig. 3.7 Furuncle in external auditory canal.

LESS COMMON LOCAL CAUSES OF EARACHE

Herpes zoster oticus and facial palsy (Fig. 3.8)

- Prodromal viraemic illness
- Headache and/or earache
- Imbalance
- May be deafness +/- tinnitus
- Vesicles on ipselateral concha and palate

Treatment

- Start oral acyclovir 400 mg five times daily for 5 days
- Discuss with ENT colleague

Bullous haemorrhagic myringitis (Fig. 3.9)

- Earache
- Red bullae on membrane

Treatment

- Analgesics. If acute otitis media supervenes, oral antibiotics may prove necessary
- Perichondritis: **REFER** urgently for in-patient management

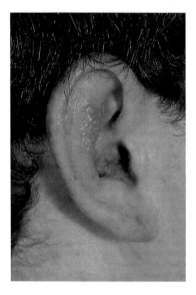

Fig. 3.8 Herpes zoster vesicles on the concha.

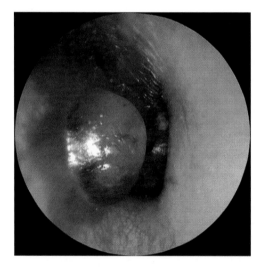

Fig. 3.9 Bullous haemorrhagic myringitis.

CAUSES OF REFERRED EARACHE

- Tonsillitis
- Glandular fever
  - Treat with simple analgesics and bedrest
  - If severe, **⟨REFER⟩** urgently for in-patient management
- Temporomandibular joint dysfunction (Fig. 3.10) occurs from malocclusion of teeth aggravated by grinding of teeth (bruxism) during sleep and associated earache without pyrexia. This may

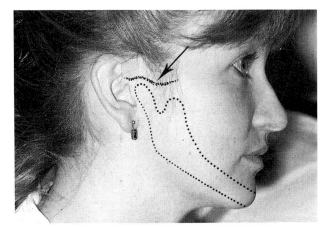

Fig. 3.10 Temperomandibular joint pain often presents as earache.

interrupt sleep; advise dental REFERRAL for assessment and night splint
- Cervical arthritis
- Tumours in mouth, throat or sinuses with their associated symptoms and signs
- Unerupted or impacted wisdom teeth: dental REFERRAL

PITFALLS

- Any unwell infant should have the ears examined to exclude acute otitis media.

- Severity of parental distress does not necessarily reflect severity of disease.

- In the management of otitis media, a 24-hour treatment just with analgesics without antibiotics is not detrimental to the outcome.

- Any recurrent purulent disease of middle or internal ear, exclude diabetes.

- Adult secretory otitis media de novo needs REFERRAL to exclude obstructive lesion of nasopharynx, e.g. carcinoma.

- Mastoid abscess must not be diagnosed in the presence of a normal or near normal tympanic membrane.

- Mastoiditis (Fig. 3.11) is part of the inflammatory process of the middle ear cleft (otitis media) and this will settle with the appropriate conservative treatment. Only when this becomes complicated as a mastoid abscess should this be REFERRED.

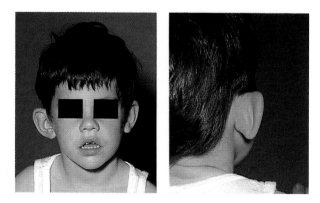

Fig. 3.11 Displacement of the pinna is a feature of acute mastoiditis.

- It is a common mistake to diagnose minimal tenderness of the adult mastoid tip as a complication of middle ear disease; tenderness over the tip (with a normal TM) is usually musculoskeletal.

- In babies the mastoid cortex is still cribriform and oedema with injection will sometimes appear as a simple extension of otitis media and should be treated as otitis media.

- Fluctuant mastoid abscess occurs behind or above the ear and may co-exist with a cholesteatoma. There is marked local and constitutional disturbance: **REFER**.

4

Ear discharge

If there is a history of previous ear surgery on the discharging ear or evidence of any surgical scarring around the ear, a detailed examination with microscope and suction is required; **REFERRAL** to the local ENT department would therefore be appropriate.

Excluding the above-mentioned group, ear discharge can occur from the following:

OTITIS EXTERNA

This is an eczematous condition of the external auditory canals ± pinna causing itch, pain and moisture (Fig. 4.1). This condition can be divided into primary and secondary.

Points of history in primary otitis externa:
- Usually bilateral
- Previous history of otitis externa, because it is often recurrent

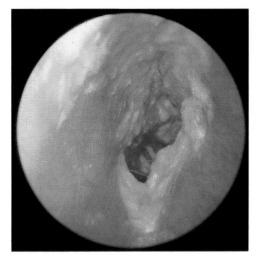

Fig. 4.1 Gross otitis externa.

- Itch is predominant although pain can be associated, occasionally severe
- Sensation of fullness because of debris accumulation
- Discharge is *not* foul-smelling
- Mild hearing loss may occur because of debris and swelling

Secondary otitis externa is usually associated with

- Middle ear disease
- Trauma, e.g. hearing aid friction
- Furuncle (see Ch. 3)
- Pseudomonas otitis externa (usually in diabetics)
- Very rarely, malignancy

MANAGEMENT OF EAR DISCHARGE

Absolute indications for REFERRAL

- Ipselateral facial palsy or other cranial nerve disorders
- True vertigo suggesting cholesteatoma
- Foul-smelling discharge suggesting cholesteatoma
- Previous ipselateral ear surgery
- CSF otorrhoea following a head injury

Treatment on the practice premises

- Initially give topical antibiotic/steroid compound drops for no more than 5 days, e.g. gentamicin/hydrocortisone.

- If the patient is diabetic, a swab should be sent off to exclude pseudomonas; if so REFER as this particular condition can be severely erosive.

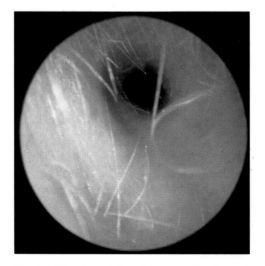

Fig. 4.2 External canal stenosis because of swollen walls.

- Advise on avoidance of shampoos, conditioners, swimming, bath water and saunas (because of excess sweat). The ear should be plugged with cotton wool pledgets smeared with petroleum jelly.

- If the above fails, repeat otoscopy which may show:

(1) Narrow canals with swollen walls (Fig. 4.2)

- Treat with glycerin and ichthammol on a ribbon gauze (Fig. 4.3)

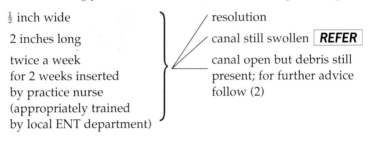

$\frac{1}{2}$ inch wide

2 inches long

twice a week
for 2 weeks inserted
by practice nurse
(appropriately trained
by local ENT department)

resolution

canal still swollen REFER

canal open but debris still
present; for further advice
follow (2)

(2) Excessive debris

treat with $\frac{1}{2}$ inch ribbon
gauze in situ for 5 days
with antibiotic installation
onto gauze or a Pope wick,
3 times a day, e.g.
gentamicin/hydrocortisone
drops

resolution

debris removed leaving
inflamed wall, use drops
for further 5 days without
gauze. If this does not
settle REFER

persistent debris REFER
for microsuction

- Any associated earache should be treated with analgesics.

- For any associated external jugular lymph node swelling or discomfort, additional treatment with oral antibiotics for 5 days is recommended.

- For itch that does not quickly respond to dressing as outlined above, an antihistamine may be useful, e.g. terfenadine, astemizole, cetirizine.

FURTHER EVALUATION

- Primary otitis externa will be seen otoscopically to have resolved by the appearance of small amounts of wax; this signifies recovery of external auditory canal epithelial function.

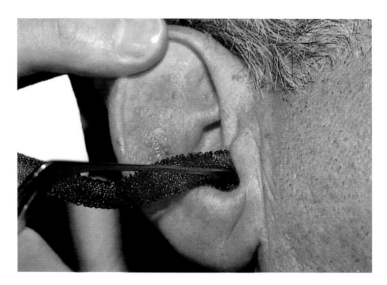

Fig. 4.3 Half-inch ribbon gauze introduced into the external canal.

- When the ear dries up, a tympanic perforation may be visible and should be sought in a case of unilateral otitis externa.

- If a perforation occurs

    – centrally (Fig. 4.4A): review after 6 weeks. If not healed, see Chapter 10.

    – in the attic (Fig. 4.4B): ‖ **REFER** ‖ because this signifies the likelihood of underlying **cholesteatoma**.

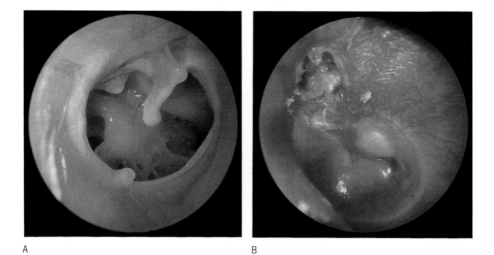

A   B

Fig. 4.4 A A total perforation in this case represents an extension of a large central perforation. **B** Attic perforation of the left tympanic membrane (at 11 o'clock position).

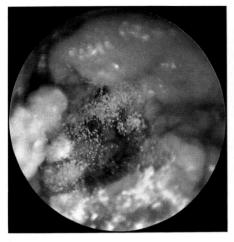
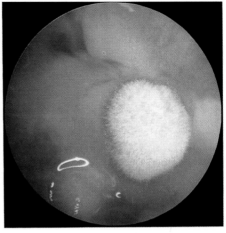

A   B

Fig. 4.5 A Spores diagnostic of a fungal infection. **B** Fungal hyphae.

PITFALLS

- Any unilateral otitis externa should have a tympanic perforation excluded. As mentioned before, a foul-smelling discharge is indicative of cholesteatoma and the patient should therefore be **REFERRED**.

- Opportunistic fungal infection (Fig. 4.5A and B), commonly *Candida* species and *Aspergillus niger*, may have occurred because of:
  - overuse of topical antibiotic drops, steroid drops or compound preparations
  - diabetes
  - general immunosuppression.

- Routine swabs from ears are unnecessary unless the patient is diabetic where pseudomonal otitis externa is more likely.

- There is a minimal risk of aminoglycoside sensorineural damage via the round window although there is little evidence of this risk in the presence of active otitis media. It is thought that protection of the inner ear is conferred by thickened inflammatory mucosa, flow of mucopus and mucosal folds during the active infection. These risks must be put into context because it must be remembered that bacterial toxins can also cause inner ear damage by diffusion across the round window; this is the medico-legal essence of the data sheet for gentamicin ear drops. The patient must be warned to stop this medication if hearing levels are affected or tinnitus occurs.

5

Childhood deafness

If a parent suspects that their child is deaf, the child should be considered deaf until otherwise proven. Overall deafness implicates bilateral hearing loss; it is unlikely that a unilateral childhood deafness presents as an overall inability to hear. A useful way of managing these children is to consider whether or not there is associated earache.

A) DEAFNESS WITHOUT EARACHE

Consider the following causes:

- Hard impacted wax; soft wax is unlikely to cause deafness

- Bilateral secretory otitis media; this may occur with or without a preceding upper respiratory tract infection

- History of pre-, peri- or postnatal complications affecting the sensorineural component

- History of meningitis or severe exanthemata should be sought but the diagnosis of deafness may well have been picked up at that time

- History of head injury with concussion

Congenital malformation of the hearing apparatus may well be associated with pinna deformity; this is usually noticed at neonatal examination.

MANAGEMENT OF PAINLESS DEAFNESS

- It is important to gain the history from the parent as to what has been noticed to arouse their suspicions of deafness in the child.

- Assess for speech and reading ability; if delayed seek full audiology and developmental assessment. This is often available via your local health visitor or even a direct service within the community from the local provider's audiology department.

- Assessment of a child's hearing can often be performed within the surgery as follows:

  Age 0–3: refer to health visitor who will liaise

  Age 3–6: the authors use Leeds Picture Discrimination cards; the method illustrated below (Fig 5.1) tests for free-field hearing which would be the most realistic for educational and social purposes

  Age 6 and over: perform a whispered voice test using easy numbers (see Fig. 6.1). Individual ear testing is useful in the older child. It should be noted that the so-called whisper is not a typical whisper but words/numbers clearly enunciated on an end-expiratory breath.

- Examination of the ear and tympanic membrane may show:

Wax and debris

- Wax may be syringed provided a perforation of tympanic membrane is not suspected (Fig. 5.2).

- Unless the wax is hard and the plug large, syringing will not cure the deafness but merely allow otoscopic examination of the membrane.

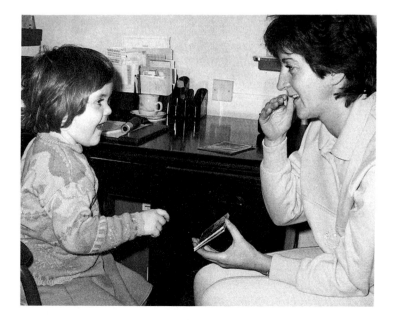

Fig. 5.1 When using Picture Discrimination Cards, the tester should use a whispered voice with the lips obscured at approximately 3 feet away from the child.

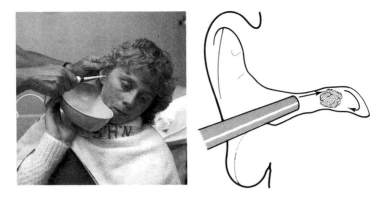

Fig. 5.2 When syringing wax, the stream of water must be directed along the roof of the external canal to avoid traumatic rupture of the tympanic membrane.

- If wax is very hard, use 5 % sodium bicarbonate drops three times a day for 5 days before further syringing.

Glue ear

This is the most likely finding diagnosed by:

- Visible blood vessels on the tympanic membrane which are often present peripherally and radially (Fig. 5.3A)
- Honey-coloured tympanic membrane (Fig. 5.3B)
- Absence of light reflex
- Blue discoloration of tympanic membrane (Fig. 5.3C)
- Presence of fluid levels (Fig. 5.3D) or air bubbles (Fig. 5.3E) behind the tympanic membrane. Handle of malleus in a horizontal position

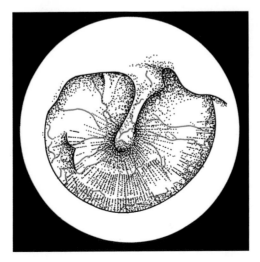

Fig. 5.3 A Radial blood vessels.

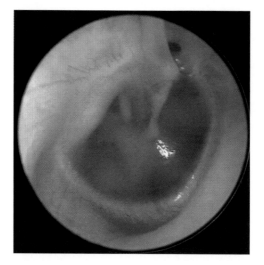

Fig. 5.3 B Honey-coloured tympanic membrane.

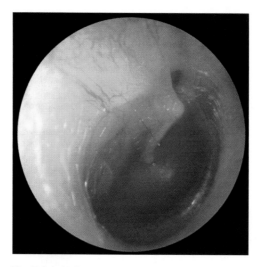

Fig. 5.3 C Air-fluid meniscus.

- Split light-reflex which indicates a retraction of the tympanic membrane. This is often found in glue ear but can also be associated with other causes of mild tympanic membrane retraction without glue (Fig. 5.3F)

When managing secretory otitis media, consider:

- The interplay between acute otitis media and secretory otitis media; each can lead one to the other.

- The basic history of speech and reading development which, if delayed, needs full audiology and developmental assessment.

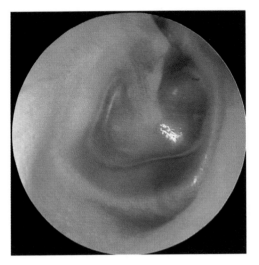

Fig. 5.3 D Dull tympanic membrane.

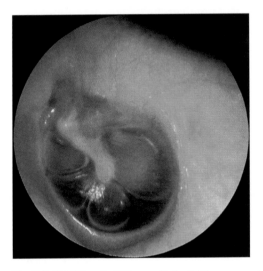

Fig. 5.3 E Bubbles of middle ear effusion in this ear were due to ototic barotrauma but similar findings can be seen in secretory otitis media.

Reduction of hearing indicates prolonged glue ear; spontaneous resolution in the near future is unlikely and we would therefore suggest ☐ **REFERRAL** ☐.

- If there is no developmental delay, observe at 2–monthly intervals to assess parental, nursery or school report of any change in hearing.

- Failure to show any improvement after the first 2 months should be considered for ☐ **REFERRAL** ☐ if education and/or social development is impaired.

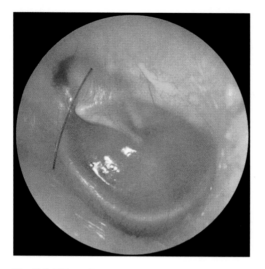

Fig. 5.3 F Tympanic retraction showing split light-reflex and horizontal malleus.

- With intermittent fluctuation of hearing, continue to observe at 2-monthly intervals.

- The older the child, the greater the likelihood of spontaneous resolution, especially after the age of 10.

- Nasal drops, oral decongestants, mucolytics and antibiotics are unlikely to help.

- Management of the parental concern in a case of glue ear is important. The confidence of the parents must be secured when considering the possibilty of a surgical intervention following failed conservative management. The authors' suggested explanation to the parents is that secretory media is an age-related condition for which grommet insertion is palliative (with regard to deafness and earache) until natural resolution occurs. Furthermore the parents should be advised that grommet insertion may need to be repeated to secure further palliation. This should not be misconstrued as failed curative attempts which unfortunately is a common but misguided belief.

- In cases of relatively asymptomatic glue ear, grommet insertion is not necessarily indicated and conservative management would therefore be logical.

- The authors recommend grommet insertion in children with socially and educationally disabling symptoms.

- It is often useful for a parent to witness an end-expiratory voice test as this will act as a reassurance or a vindication of their concerns. If the response to such testing is unsatisfactory, then more formal audiological testing should be requested.

Tympanic perforation: **REFER** for further assessment

DEAFNESS WITH EARACHE

Consider:

- Acute otitis media (Fig. 5.4) often preceded by an upper respiratory tract infection
- Hard impacted wax

MANAGEMENT OF PAINFUL DEAFNESS

- Treat as acute otitis earache (see Ch. 3): 12–24 h of a paediatric paracetamol preparation in appropriate maximum doses.

- Beyond 24 h: give a 3-day course of a maximum dose of antibiotic appropriate for the patient's age.

- A spontaneous discharge from the affected ear will relieve pain but a secretory otitis media (glue ear) may supervene and the cycle will be restarted once the acute perforation has healed.

- If earache settles but deafness persists, treat as deafness without earache.

- Nose drops do not contribute.

- Repeated episodes are worth tackling with low dose regimes of trimethoprim (see Ch. 3) although **REFERRAL** may be necessary if this is unsuccessful.

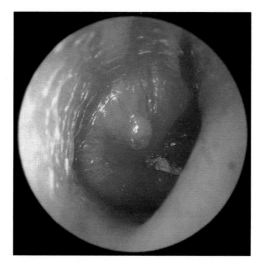

Fig. 5.4 Acute otitis media with characteristic bulging tympanic membranes.

PITFALLS

- If the parent or guardian feels their child is deaf and the ears and membranes are both normal, suspect underlying sensorineural deafness and REFER .

- In a child deaf with secretory otitis media, do remember that a sensorineural deafness may also be present. This should be borne in mind especially with a markedly deaf child: REFER .

6

Adult deafness

This is normally of slower onset and the patient will have socially inadequate hearing with bilateral deafness; unilateral hearing loss causes a more specific deafness, for example, on the telephone or with direction of voice at a business meeting and is unlikely to have an impact on free-field hearing.

POINTS OF HISTORY

- Previous ear surgery
- Childhood illness (exanthemata) sometimes involves a sensorineural loss as well as a conductive loss
- Head injury
- Severe systemic illness and ototoxic drugs
- Occupational history may give a story of prolonged noise exposure
- Hobbies, such as rifle shooting (usually over many years) may suggest this as a contributory cause
- Family history of deafness suggests otosclerosis or familial sensorineural deafness

FINDINGS THAT CAN BE MANAGED IN THE SURGERY

Wax may produce a more acute history of deafness. In the absence of a history of perforation or previous ear operation, 5% sodium bicarbonate drops can be administered for 5 days, followed by syringing. Prolonged use of OTC (over the counter) drops may well cause a chemical otitis externa.

TESTING THE HEARING IN THE SURGERY

- Whispered voice; assessment at 3 feet distance by masking the contralateral ear (Fig. 6.1)

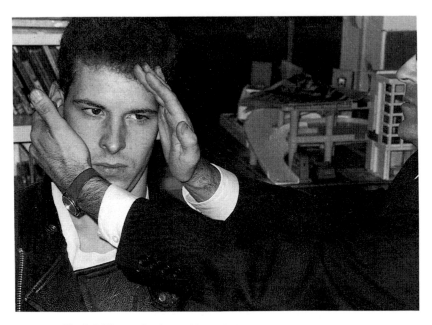

Fig. 6.1 When performing a whispered voice test, ensure that the patient's eyes are shielded to preventing lipreading. The opposite tragus is lightly rubbed to prevent the sound being heard by the other ear.

- Conversational voice at 3 feet distance from each ear with gentle tragal rubbing of untested ear to prevent crossover of sound

- General conversational voice with lips obscured from patient's view

- Tuning fork tests: quite helpful although wide variation makes really accurate diagnosis impossible

  - Weber and Rinne tests (Fig. 6.2) to distinguish between conductive deafness and sensorineural deafness. A 512-Hz tuning fork is recommended; higher frequencies fade too frequently and lower frequencies cause excessive vibration

- An interrupted pure-tone audiogram (as opposed to a sweep test): useful if available (see Ch. 7). This may be undertaken at the hospital or indeed commissioned at the practice

FURTHER MANAGEMENT WITHIN THE PRACTICE SETTING

Symmetrical bilateral sensorineural deafness in the over 50s is very likely to be due to **presbycusis**. The GP should ascertain the specific situations with which the patient is having difficulties:

- Telephone or door bell; these can be remedied via the appropriate telecommunication provider

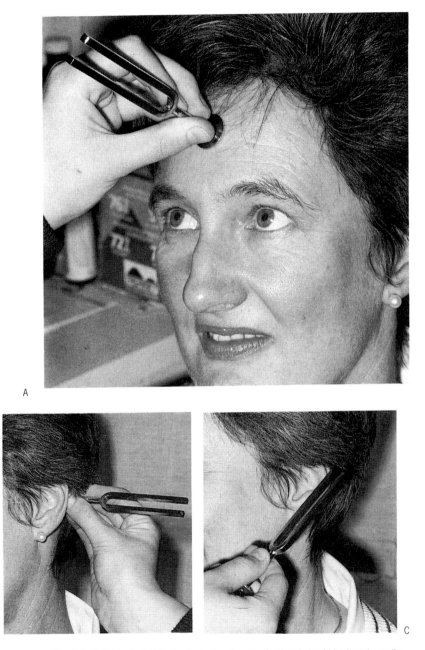

Fig. 6.2 A Weber test. A tuning fork placed on the forehead should be heard equally in both ears. If the sound is heard better in one ear, either (i) that ear may have a conductive deafness or (ii) the other ear has a sensorineural (nerve) deafness. **B** Rinne test. The tuning fork is placed on the mastoid process behind the ear. The patient indicates when the sound is no longer heard. **C** The fork is then held adjacent to the ear. The fork can still be heard when the ear is normal, or when the ear has a sensorineural deafness. In a conductive loss, the sound is heard better behind the ear than adjacent to it.

● Hearing in crowded surroundings; an aid is not helpful in fil-
tering out this distraction (this is a central function) and this
limitation must be made quite clear to the patient if an aid is
prescribed. Lip-reading skills are often more helpful in a noisy
working environment. An aid is optimal for augmenting communication in a relatively quiet environment.

The local audiology department is likely to have a protocol for
direct referral in the above circumstances and avoids an unnecessary referral to the ENT department.

WHEN TO REFER AND TO WHOM

● If a patient is disabled by a hearing deficit, management should
be advised appropriate to social and occupational disability.
There is likely to be a protocol-based direct access facility at the
local community or hospital audiology department; their
audiometry results may include advice for specialist referral if
there is conductive or asymmetrical sensorineural loss.

● Conductive deafness of unknown cause (see Ch. 7) should be
REFERRED for further assessment to ascertain the diagnosis
and management options.

● All sudden deafness should be REFERRED if wax is not visible.

● Asymmetrical sensorineural deafness **over 10 decibels** in the
otherwise healthy individual should be REFERRED to exclude
the rare diagnosis of **acoustic neuroma**.

PITFALLS

● Even if malingering is suspected in relation to an industrial
or criminal claim, this should be REFERRED for audiology
testing.

7

Pure tone audiometry – nature and interpretation

A pure tone audiogram (PTA) is a chart showing hearing levels (measured in decibels) at various frequencies (measured in cycles per sound or hertz) (Fig. 7.1).

The vertical scale of decibels is logarithmic; that is to say, if two sounds differ by 20 decibels, the difference between them in intensity will be 10^2 or 100-fold. Likewise if the difference between

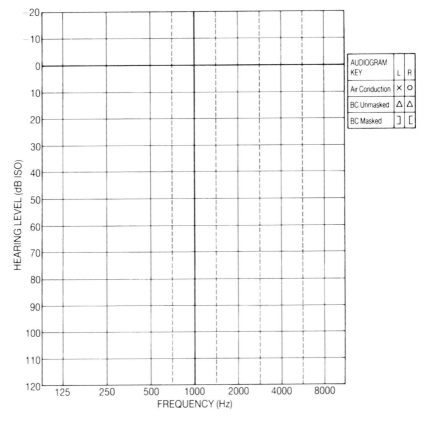

Fig. 7.1 Pure tone audiogram.

those two sounds is 30 decibels, the difference in intensity will be 10^3 or 1000-fold, etc.

The audiographic scales are based on a population average: e.g. 10 decibels means better than the population average of 0 decibels.

Each frequency is specifically tested for:

- Air conduction via ear phones. This measures sound levels heard via the normal processes, i.e. a sound wave which hits the tympanic membrane which is then transmitted along the ossicles to the inner ear and the electrical pathways systems, i.e. cochlea and auditory nerve.

- Bone conduction via a transducer applied to the mastoid bone. (A masking noise has to be applied to the ear which is not being tested.) This reflects the ability of the electrical systems of the ear to sense and transduce sound, i.e. the function of the cochlea and auditory nerve.

Deafness can be divided into two catergories:

- Conductive loss
- Sensorineural (cochlear-nerve) loss

CONDUCTIVE LOSS

This represents a loss of sound in the conduction system of the ear between the tympanic membrane and cochlea (via the ossicles). Reduction of hearing can therefore occur with:

- Glue ear
- Large perforations
- Dislocation, destruction or adhesion of the ossicles

The audiogram shows a normal sensorineural (nerve) pattern but a reduced conductive hearing pattern as below (Fig. 7.2).

SENSORINEURAL LOSS

This represents a defect within the electrical aspect of the ear, i.e. cochlea and auditory nerve. The audiogram (Fig. 7.3) shows reduced levels for both air conduction and bone conduction.

Presbycusis

Hearing loss with age is a variant of a sensorineural hearing loss but mainly occurs initially at high frequencies (Fig. 7.4).

Mixed losses are also commonly found, e.g. presbycusis on top of longstanding middle ear disease such as tympanosclerotic scarring (Fig. 7.5).

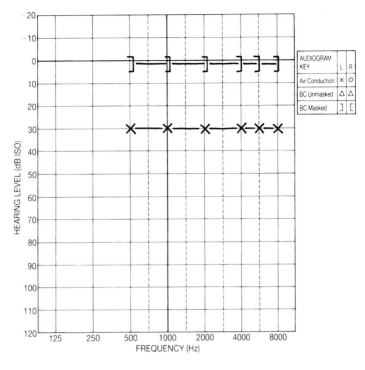

Fig. 7.2 Pure tone audiogram

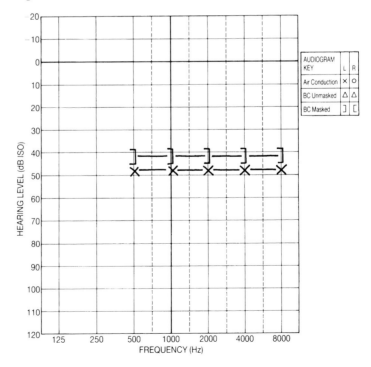

Fig. 7.3 Pure tone audiogram

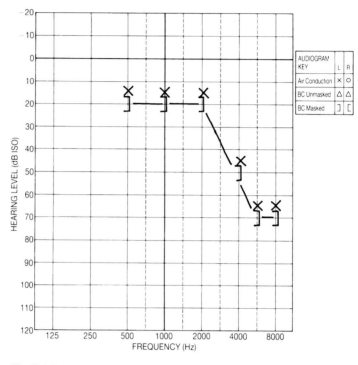

Fig. 7.4 Pure tone audiogram

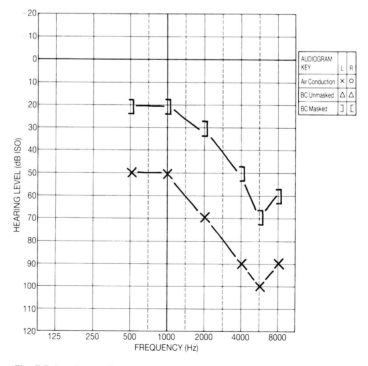

Fig. 7.5 Pure tone audiogram

8

Services for patients with impaired hearing

These services are practically subdivided between children and adults because their requirements are clearly different.

CHILDREN

Once it is established that a child has sensorineural or irreversibly conductive deafness, a referral is made to a teacher for the deaf who will help plan educational development, auditory training and arrange for the fitting of a hearing aid if appropriate. There is a close communication between:

- Parents
- Local ENT department
- Local audiology clinic
- Primary health care team
- Educational psychologists

The child's education is planned from an early age as soon as chronic deafness is diagnosed so that competence in communication is achieved by the age of 5 years.

Education

- *Normal schools* are attended by 50% of children who have irreversible deafness and are visited by teachers of the deaf. These teachers help and advise on:
  - Use of hearing aids
  - Help with lip reading
  - Assessment of the child's progress
- *Special units* are situated in some schools and, indeed, there is now a trend away from recommending schools for the deaf. These units offer:
  - Induction loop aids which amplify the teacher's voice; in turn this is picked up by the child's hearing aid.

- Radio-hearing aids which comprise a radio-microphone which is hand-held by the teacher. The radio-microphone transmits to a radio-receiver worn by the child.

- *Schools for the deaf* are still part of the education system although the trend is towards special units within normal schools.

- *Additional skills* include manual communication known as 'signing'. These manual skills are combined with oral communication to form 'total communication'.

ADULTS

A reflex prescription for a hearing aid does not necessarily meet the need of the patient who may well relegate the aid to a drawer! A thorough history is vital in order to reveal the specific circumstances of hearing difficulty, e.g. doorbells, shopping, crossing roads. It should also be remembered that a change of job or working environment can reveal a hitherto unnoticed hearing difficulty.

Limitation awareness

The clinician must be aware of the patient's *ideas, concerns* and *expectations* of this hearing loss. Such consultation skills will enable patients to develop the necessary knowledge and insight around their difficulties and thus 'cross the bridge' and overcome fears to manage their problem successfully. Examples of such situations would be:

- The newly presenting middle-aged patient with a mild loss audiometrically who experiences difficulties only in the presence of background noise; it is not enough to explain that a hearing aid would not be beneficial and merely amplify all noise but that this is a problem of *auditory discrimination* rather than *auditory threshhold*. A far more effective approach would be to develop behavioural changes and lip-reading skills, the attitude to which must be destigmatised from the association with very severe deafness. It should also be advised that the patient is addressed with clarity of diction rather than sheer volume.

- The older, perhaps retired patient with socially embarrassing presbycusis which also may threaten safety at the roadside etc. There may be a fearful recall of severe parental deafness and a secret awareness of poor hearing prognosis. This fear should be acknowledged but be dealt with positively by highlighting the benefits of a coordinated approach using hearing aids, lip-reading skills and domestic devices. It should be remembered that other sensory and motor modalities should be evaluated, e.g. vision, hand arthritis in manipulating aids etc.

- The young adult who has recently started in a new working or student environment with a perceived deafness which may have been originally suggested by a peer or someone of authority. Audiometric results may well be normal! This perceived deafness is most likely associated with anxieties related to the challenge of the new environment. Reassurance is vital.

Hearing aids

These are subdivided into *ear level* and *bone conductor*. It must be remembered that hearing aids are merely amplifiers not discriminators of sound. Unscrambling from ambient distracting sound is largely a CNS function and, again, is not accommodated by a hearing aid.

- Ear level aids can be further subdivided into *'in the ear'* (ITE) (Fig. 8.1) and *post-aural* (Fig. 8.2). The ITE aids are commercially available either from the high street or through licensed NHS audiology departments as a private purchase. The NHS normally provide post-aural aids via the local audiology department. Recent additions, available privately, are ITE aids which attempt to filter out background noise but these are still under evaluation.

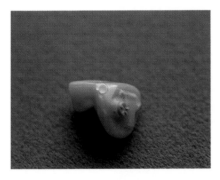

Fig. 8.1 In the ear hearing aid.

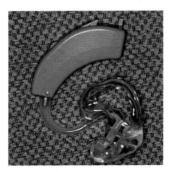

Fig. 8.2 Post-aural hearing aid.

● Bone conductor aids (Fig. 8.3) are reserved for the profoundly deaf; the aid will provide auditory and vibro-tactile input. Chronic otitis media or severe externa may preclude the use of an ear level aid, in which case a bone conductor will be a useful alternative.

Domestic devices

These improve communication for the deaf and include modifications to:

● Telephones

(a) Bell	– extension bells
	– flashing lights
	– amplified bells, buzzers and hooters
(b) Handset	– amplification
	– adjustable volume control
	– induction couplers within the handset will amplify sound in the hearing aid when it is set in the 'T' position (Fig. 8.4)

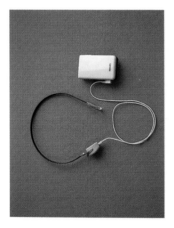

Fig. 8.3 Bone conductor hearing aid.

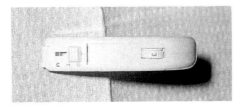

Fig. 8.4 Hearing aids have an OTM switch. O is off, M is the normal operating position and T is used in combination with induction loop mechanisms. The volume control is numbered 1 to 4.

- Television
  - Separate loudspeakers
  - Induction loops which generate an electromagnetic field; this in turn generates a current and signal in the hearing aid when set in the 'T' position. This facility is available in some cinemas and auditoria.
  - Ceefax and Oracle offer subtitles and specific services for the deaf

USEFUL ADDRESSES

Royal National Institute for the Deaf
19–23 Featherstone Street
London EC1Y 8SL
Tel: 0171 296–8000

Link
British Centre for Deafened People
19 Hartfield Road
Eastbourne
East Sussex BR21 2AR
Tel: 01323 638230
(This organisation is particularly useful for the suddenly deafened)

City Lit Centre for Deaf People & Speech Therapy (adults)
Keeley House
Keeley Street
London WC2B 4BA
Tel: 0171 430–0548

9

Tinnitus

Tinnitus is a descriptive term applied to noises either in the ear or head. Patients will often describe the noise as a whistling kettle although some will describe a pulsatile quality synchronous with the heartbeat. Tinnitus can be considered as subjective or objective.

SUBJECTIVE TINNITUS

This is often secondary to sensorineural auditory defects. It can be exacerbated by the middle ear disease which prevents ambient masking sound from reaching the inner ear.

Many adult patients are extremely anxious about their *subjective* tinnitus in case it represents sinister disease such as a brain tumour; appropriate reassurance will be required. Tinnitus intensity will vary according to levels of anxiety because of a fear of inexorable worsening; the patient should be strongly reassured that this is not the case and that tinnitus tends to settle back to previous levels once anxiety has been addressed.

Most patients with subjective tinnitus will give a history of deafness:

- If the deafness is socially embarrassing, **REFER** for audiology and aiding, which may well quell the tinnitus as well as relieve deafness.

- If the tinnitus is mild, explain that tinnitus represents the ravages of 'wear and tear' on the inner ear. This reassurance may well reduce the element of anxiety with consequent reduction in tinnitus.

- If the patient is struggling to cope with tinnitus, then the help of a psychologist (either in-house or via the local hospital) is advised. Behavioural management is vital if the patient is to accommodate the tinnitus successfully.

51

- Tinnitus maskers producing white noise can be offered via the local audiology department but only in conjunction with overall behaviour management.

- Those who are greatly troubled may well benefit from contact with the Tinnitus Association.

- Patients with tympanic abnormalities should be REFERRED to the local ENT department for thorough assessment.

- Children occasionally complain of *subjective* tinnitus; secretory otitis media is often the cause (see Ch. 5).

OBJECTIVE TINNITUS

This is when the noise is actually heard by other people standing nearby. This is very rare and should be REFERRED to exclude vascular abnormalities.

PITFALLS

- Medications for tinnitus per se are unhelpful. It may be appropriate to use psychotropic drugs if secondary agitation and depression occur.

- Asymmetrical sensorineural hearing loss may present as a unilateral tinnitus and should be REFERRED to exclude the rare diagnosis of acoustic neuroma.

USEFUL ADDRESSES

British Tinnitus Association
Room 6
14–18 West Bar Green
Sheffield
S2 2DA

R.N.I.D. Tinnitus Helpline
2 Pelham Court
Pelham Road
Nottingham
NG5 1AP

10

Tympanic perforations

Tympanic membrane perforations can be managed in general practice by considering whether they are:

- Attic perforations (Fig. 10.1A)
- Central perforations (Fig. 10.1B)

ATTIC PERFORATIONS

These are diagnosed by:

- Otoscopic detection of a superiorly placed small perforation ± granulation tissue ± visible cholesteatoma

- Attic perforations are usually associated with a cholesteatoma and often suspected by inference, i.e. a foul-smelling discharge and debris which obscures a clear view of the tympanic

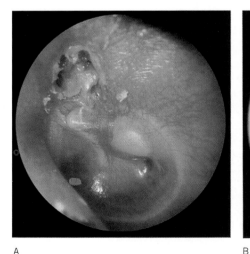 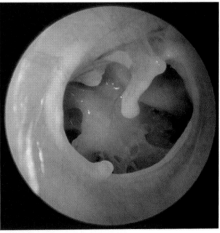

A   B

Fig. 10.1 A Attic perforation of the left tympanic membrane (at 11 o'clock position). **B** A total perforation in this case represents an extension of a large central perforation.

membrane. The discharge is usually from secondary *proteus* and *pseudomonas* infection of the cholesteatoma itself.

The presenting symptoms and conditions caused by cholesteatoma (Fig. 10.2) are:

- Deafness
- Foul otorrhoea
- Earache
- Ipselateral facial palsy
- Vertigo
- Abscess over mastoid bone
- Meningitis

Management

- All suspected attic perforations or cholesteatoma should be **REFERRED** for microscopy and possible surgery.

CENTRAL PERFORATIONS

- Can be safely observed for a period by the GP
- Occurring in response to trauma or otitis media may well heal spontaneously

Management

- If the tympanic membrane is obscured by purulent discharge, then prescribe at most a 5–day course of antibiotic ear drops.
- There is a minimal risk of aminoglycoside sensorineural damage via the round window although there is little evidence of this risk in the presence of active otitis media. It is thought that protection of the inner ear is conferred by thickened inflam-

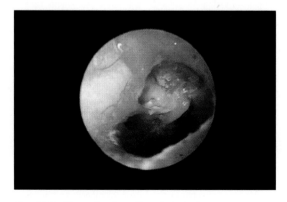

Fig. 10.2 Attic perforation with a cholesteatoma.

matory mucosa, flow of mucopus and mucosal folds during the active infection. These risks must be put into context because it must be remembered that bacterial toxins can also cause inner ear damage by diffusion across the round window; this is the medico-legal essence of the data sheet for gentamicin ear drops. The patient should be warned to stop this medication if hearing levels are affected or tinnitus occurs.

- When the perforation is dry, then observe and advise the patient to prevent water entering the ear by use of cottonwool smeared with petroleum jelly. Review the patient in 6 weeks; thereafter, the patient should report back with any further trouble.

- Unilateral dry central perforations do not usually interfere with free-field hearing provided that the other ear is hearing normally.

- If deafness with a central perforation is severe, consider ossicular disruption or scarring; again if unilateral this should not impact on free-field hearing.

INDICATIONS FOR REFERRAL

- Recurrent otorrhoea
- Earache from secondary otitis externa
- Deafness
- Troublesome vertigo due to the caloric effect of cold air
- Occupational necessity for intact tympanic membranes, e.g. armed forces, hobbies, etc.

Should a symptomless central perforation persist, the GP can confidently reassure the patient that no active treatment is required, except protecting the ear from bath and swimming-pool water, etc.

PITFALLS

- If a perforation occurs as a result of criminal assault, it would be as well to obtain an audiogram at initial presentation, as well as after 6 weeks, by which time spontaneous healing will have taken place.

- Central perforations are themselves painless; pain would suggest secondary otitis externa from discharge spilling into the deep part of the external auditory canal.

11

Dizziness, giddiness and vertigo

- These are often the patient's words to describe his predicament. The GP must therefore assess the history to ascertain whether symptoms are of true vertigo.

- Vertigo is specifically a hallucination of rotatory movement. The history from the patient must indicate a definite sensation of spinning; this is crucial.

- If the history does not include spinning but rather light-headedness, this particular symptom calls for a general medical assessment.

- If the symptom of vertigo is convincing, then the general practitioner has to assess whether the origin is:

  - Otogenic
  - CNS.

OTOGENIC

(1) Ménière's syndrome

This is all too frequently diagnosed because it is assumed to be synonymous with recurrent vertigo and deafness. Ménière's syndrome represents an idiopathic endolymphatic hydrops where the endolymph channel of the inner ear is expanded relative to the perilymph channels. To diagnose Ménière's syndrome, the following symptom complex should present:

- Vertigo and nausea
- Change of hearing directly associated with the episodes of spinning
- Sense of fullness or blocking of the ear
- Tinnitus classically appears to change its usual pitch in relation to the episodes of spinning
- Clustering of attacks

- These various elements developed and resolved virtually together as a paroxysmal episode.

Management

- **REFER** for assessment and confirmation of the diagnosis as treatment may subsequently be lifelong.
- There is a great variation in modes of treatment for this condition and we suggest that each patient will require a management plan which is arrived at by communication between GP, hospital consultant and patient.
- Possible drug treatments include labyrinthine sedatives and betahistine which is thought to have some action on the inner fluid dynamics.
- Excessive dietary salt and liquid intake should be curbed.

(2) Viral labyrinthitis

Key points

- Recent viral URTI
- Associated nausea or vomiting
- No associated loss of hearing necessarily
- Normal tympanic membrane
- History starting with true vertigo and usually modifying into a sense of general imbalance before complete resolution

Management

- Reassurance that it is self-limiting in a few weeks, occasionally months
- Advise patients to remain in bed if necessary
- Normal activities to be curtailed
- Labyrinthine sedatives; if vomiting precludes the oral route, use suppositories, parenteral administration or buccal preparation
- If persistent over 6 weeks **REFER**

(3) Benign positional vertigo

Key points

- Fleeting vertigo usually when the patient lies down with head in triggering position (usually one particular ear towards the pillow)
- Vertigo can be elicited in the surgery by lying patient on a couch with head (supported by clinician's hand) over the top edge,

with one ear lowermost. The patient is instructed to sit up quickly and fix a stare ahead; nystagmus associated with resulting vertigo may be seen for a few seconds. The process, known as the Hallpike manoeuvre, is reversed to elicit nystagmus again. It is the downmost ear which is responsible; the fault is thought to be loose otolith gravel in the posterior semicircular canal of the labyrinth.

- Normal or 'non-acute' tympanic membranes

Management

- Give reassurance that this is usually self-limiting over a few weeks.

- Advise patient to remain in the triggering position for as long as possible until vertigo has settled, rather than 'escape'. This will improve central compensation and may encourage a loose ampullary otolith to stabilise.

- Labyrinthine sedatives may not be wholly successful but are worth a try.

- If persistent beyond 3 months or particularly severe, **REFER** to the local ENT out-patient department for otolith repositioning techniques such as the Epley manoeuvre.

CENTRAL NERVOUS SYSTEM ORIGIN

(1) Vertebro-basilar insufficiency

Key points

- Association with neck extension and rotation
- Normal tympanic membranes
- Associated neck pain related to underlying cervical spondylitis
- Possibly generalised features of arteriosclerosis, e.g. bruits, claudication
- Occasional TIA symptoms

Management

- Cervical collar
- Reappraisal of life-style
- Specific treatment of osteoarthritis if applicable

(2) Acoustic neuroma

This is rare but should be suspected with any vague sense of imbalance associated with a persistent unilateral tinnitus and deafness. In extreme cases, fifth and seventh cranial nerves can be subtly involved; REFER .

In general URGENT REFERRAL is necessary when vertigo is associated with:

- Attic cholesteatoma
- Ear discharge
- Deafness
- Facial palsy
- Headaches and neurological abnormalities, e.g. PICA (posterior inferior cerebellar artery) syndrome, incipient hydrocephalus
- Previous ear surgery
- Recent head injury

Following ENT specialist investigation and treatment, a number of patients may have conditions manageable thereafter by the general practitioner:

- Ménière's syndrome
- Vertebro-basilar insufficiency
- Neurological conditions
- Financially-motivated compensation-associated conditions

Consider involving physiotherapists to palliate persistent and non advancing vertigo.

FISTULA TEST

In cases of attic cholesteatoma with or without ear discharge, it is quite possible for the lateral semicircular canal of the labyrinth to be eroded. In such cases of cholesteatoma and a history of vertigo, the fistula test may well confirm this scenario but not always. The method is simple; the clinician presses the external meatus of the affected ear by pressing the tragus. The patient will immediately have vertigo and the eyes will turn away to the good side; when the finger pressure is removed, the eyes will return to the centre followed by a brief nystagmus.

PITFALLS

- Patients with loss of consciousness associated with vertigo should be REFERRED for a neurological opinion.

- Light-headedness should also be asked for specifically. Remember that both symptoms of vertigo and light-headedness may coexist and should be unravelled from the history.

- Presbycusis and presbystasis are common problems in the elderly. A history of light-headedness only will **exclude** conditions such as Ménière's syndrome. Even if there is a genuine history of vertigo from, say, vertebro-basilar insufficiency, the co-existance of unrelated presbycusis does not constitute Ménière's syndrome.

- Blood pressure measurement should be taken as part of the initial examination as balance disturbance can be an initial presentation of hypertension.

12

Facial palsy

This is classified as:

- Upper motor neurone; this spares the ipselateral frontalis muscle and is commonly part of a cerebrovascular accident or neurogenic disease.

- Lower motor neurone; this involves the ipselateral frontalis muscle along with the other ipselateral facial muscles (Fig. 12.1) innervated by the seventh cranial nerve.

In the ENT field, the lower motor neurone lesion is the more usual and the following diagnoses should therefore be considered:

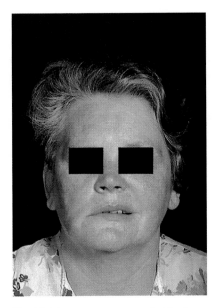

Fig. 12.1 Lower motor neurone facial palsy.

BELL'S PALSY

This is a diagnosis of exclusion.

- 75 % fully recover in 3 weeks; failure of resolution after 3 weeks should prompt a **REFERRAL**. The likely explanation of delayed resolution is degeneration of some or all of the facial nerve fibres.

- May be preceded by pain around the ipselateral ear.

- Patients may well present to the GP fearful that they are having a stroke.

- Taste fibres in the trigeminal nerve accompany sensory branches to the anterior two-thirds of the tongue; taste and lacrimation recover early.

Management

- Management of patients' morale in respect of their expectations especially if recovery does not occur quickly.

- ACTH and steroids have not proven to be beneficial.

- The eye should be protected in the early stages with artificial tear drops and eyepad, especially when the patient is outdoors or asleep.

- If secondary corneal damage is suspected, **REFER** to ophthalmologist.

- Slowly resolving cases should be sent for transcutaneous nerve stimulation by an appropriate physiotherapy department to prevent facial muscular contracture.

- Alternative neurological diagnosis should be considered in cases with multiple neuropathies.

HERPES ZOSTER

Shingles can affect the ipselateral auricular skin, palate and pharynx as well as the facial nerve. The acoustic nerve may also be affected; this scenario is also known as Ramsay-Hunt syndrome. Even the smallest vesicle on the ipselateral concha or palate will be diagnostic (Fig 12.2).

Management

It would probably be as well to discuss the management with the local specialist department with a view to admission for:

- Analgesics

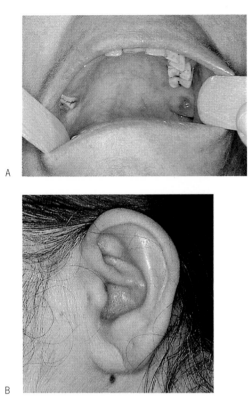

Fig. 12.2 A In Ramsay-Hunt syndrome herpes zoster vesicles can be seen on the ipselateral half of the palate. A tooth has been removed in the mistaken diagnosis of decay; it was the prodromal pain in the palate and gum of Ramsay-Hunt syndrome. A palatal rash subsequently developed. **B** herpes zoster vesicles on the concha.

- Acyclovir orally or intravenously
- Corneal protection (especially during sleep) using eyepad and hypomellose eye drops ('artificial tears')
- Electroneurographic (ENG) assessment of the seventh nerve
- Management of patients' morale in respect of their expectations because facial recovery may not occur

ADVANCING MIDDLE EAR DISEASE

If a lower motor neurone facial palsy occurs in association with an ipselateral otorrhoea or identifiable cholesteatoma, **REFER**.

POST-TRAUMATIC CASES

These will probably present to the Accident and Emergency Department, although an occasional patient will present to the GP's surgery and should be **REFERRED** to the ENT department forthwith.

13

Nasal blockage

This is the sensation of reduced air flow, either unilaterally or bilaterally. The basic subdivisions are:

- Mucosal swelling due to:
  - coryza
  - allergic rhinitis
  - vasomotor rhinitis (syn non-allergic)
  - polypi
- Septal deviation
  - of traumatic origin
  - idiopathic
- Valvular inspiratory collapse at one or both nostrils
- Nasopharyngeal obstruction from
  - enlarged adenoids
  - polypi
  - tumour

ASSOCIATED POINTS OF THE HISTORY

The differential diagnosis of mucosal swelling is often discernable by the swelling.

Allergic rhinitis

Key points

- Itch of
  - palate
  - eyes
  - nose
  - throat
- Sneezing
- Watery nasal discharge

A searching history is needed to identify culpable allergens, e.g.

- House dust and house dust mite
- Pollens of grasses, trees, flowers
- Feathers and down
- Moulds and spores
- Animal dander

A nasal challenge would be ideal but may precipitate an allergic crisis and would therefore not be appropriate in a general practice setting. A RAST (radioallergoimmunosorbent test) on a sample of venous blood is now commonly available via the local pathology laboratory and can be tailored according to suspected allergens from the history.

A skin test is less specific and measures a dermal rather than a nasal response.

The symptoms of allergic rhinitis may be indistinguishable from vasomotor rhinitis.

Vasomotor rhinitis

This is exacerbated by:

- Perfume
- Aerosol sprays
- Change in air temperature
- Tobacco smoke and other pollutants

Note also:

- Itch is not usually present.
- Sides of blockage may alternate.
- Vasomotor and allergic rhinitis may coexist.
- Onset may be associated with hormonal changes of puberty and menopause.
- Onset may be associated with anxiety and frustration; it is said that children cry through their eyes and adults through their noses!

Nasal polypi

These produce a more steady development of symptoms and may be an extension of allergic or vasomotor rhinitis and often compounded by ethmoidal congestion. Also the patient may have experienced:

- Previous polypectomies
- Diminution or loss of sense of smell

ALLERGIC AND VASOMOTOR RHINITIS

Findings

- Swollen inferior turbinates (Fig. 13.1)
- Pale or mauve-coloured inferior turbinates
- Excessively moist nasal mucosa
- Allergic crease from repeated allergic 'salutes' which are more obvious in young people (Fig. 13.2)
- Reduced nasal airway

To distinguish between allergic and vasomotor rhinitis, the history is often more helpful than relying on specific physical findings.

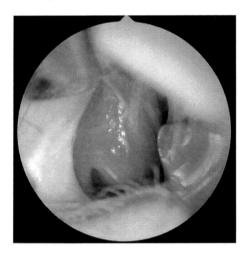

Fig. 13.1 Swollen inferior turbinates are often a cause of nasal blockage because of their allergic and non-allergic mucosal congestion.

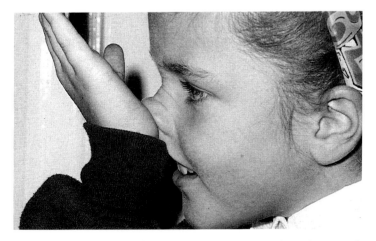

Fig. 13.2 Persistent rubbing of the nose to alleviate the discomfort and momentarily improve the airflow will eventually cause a crease of the skin on the nasal bridge.

Initial therapies

(1) Topical medications

Treatment of choice:
- Intranasal aqueous steroid sprays, e.g. beclomethasone, budesonide, flunisolide, fluticasone

- Avoidance advice concerning likely allergens

- If nasal drip predominates, topical anticholinergic spray such as ipratropium may be helpful

(2) Oral treatment

We have found oral medications to be more useful in supporting topical intranasal treatment. In cases of residual nasal or additional extranasal symptoms, then oral medications can be strongly recommended:

- Antihistamines, e.g. astemizole, terfenadine, loratidine
- Pseudoephedrine may help in vasomotor rhinitis
- Combination preparations combining an antihistamine and a sympathomimetic

(3) Inhalation

- Steam (not directly from kettle)
- Menthol
- Tinct benzoin

These inhalations reduce discomfort of nasal blockage and can be taken for a few minutes every 2 hours.

(4) Surgical intervention

Surgery to reduce the size of the inferior turbinates is strongly advised when:

- Blockage is severe
- Medical treatment fails

Surgical reduction of inferior turbinates will improve both patency and access for future topical intranasal steroids.

GP MANAGEMENT OF NASAL POLYPI

- If symptoms are mild, intranasal steroid drops, e.g. beclomethasone (Betnesol drops), should be applied twice a day with the head in the extended position. Regular steroid sprays may be preferred and worth trying as an alternative to drops. Smoking should be discouraged.

- If pus is visible it would be prudent to take a bacteriology swab and start empirically on metronidazole and penicillin for 7 days prior to intranasal steroids.

- Nasal polyps often recur and in such cases the patient will require maintenance intranasal steroid spray and occasional oral steroid pulses (Fig. 13.3).

  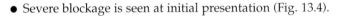 **REFER** when:

- Medical management fails; it should be borne in mind that, in many cases of nasal polyposis, surgery is an adjunct to long-term medical management of what is basically a chronic rhino-sinopathy.

- Severe blockage is seen at initial presentation (Fig. 13.4).

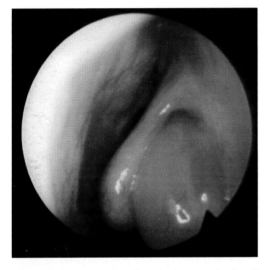

Fig. 13.3 Endoscopic view of nasal polyp emerging from the meatus below the middle turbinate.

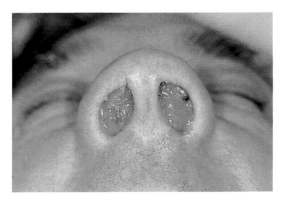

Fig. 13.4 Nasal polyps usually arise from the middle meatus.

- Neoplasm is suspected by the presence of a unilateral polyp with or without bleeding.

SEPTAL DEVIATION

May be associated with:

- External deformity of either the nasal bridge or nasal tip or, indeed, both (Fig. 13.5)
- A history of trauma, although not necessarily so
- Unilateral blockage as a presenting symptom
- Any of the aforementioned mucosal abnormalities

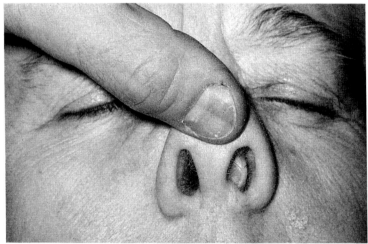

A

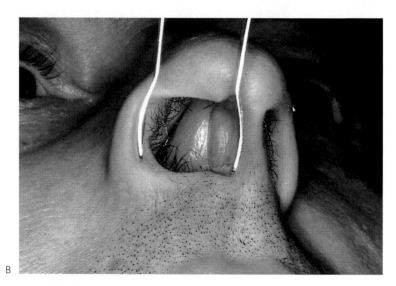

B

Fig. 13.5 The septal cartilage can be deviated at **A** the front or **B** the middle.

Findings

- Tilting the nasal tip upwards the clinician may reveal a deviation anteriorly. Deviations posteriorly will be seen through an auriscope with a large speculum.

- Reduced unilateral flow (see Fig. 2.5).

Management

- If blockage is solely due to septal deviation: REFER .

- If overlying allergic or non-allergic rhinitis, topical steroid sprays may just prove sufficient; if not REFER .

VALVULAR INSPIRATORY COLLAPSE

A minor degree of valvular movement of the nostrils during inspiration is physiologically normal. When excessive, the patient will present with nasal blockage on inspiration (Fig. 13.6); REFER .

NASOPHARYNGEAL BLOCKAGE

Causes of obstruction:

- Enlarged adenoids in children
- Antrochoanal polyp hanging into nasopharynx; this type of polyp is usually solitary
- Tumours

Management of suspected nasopharyngeal blockage

- If adenoids are thought to be responsible , request a lateral X-ray of the nasopharynx. If the air shadow is thicker than the soft palate shadow, adenoid enlargement is unlikely to be a major

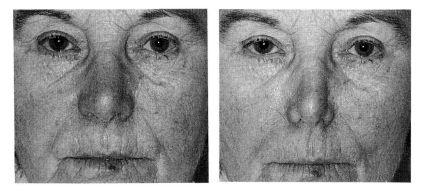

Fig. 13.6 Pronounced sucking in of the alae (nostrils) on inspiration reduces the airflow.

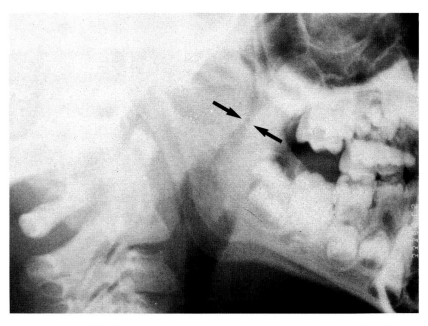

Fig. 13.7 The arrows show that the nasopharynx has an air shadow which is thinner than the soft palate; adenoid enlargement is the usual cause in children.

contribution to the blockage; if the air shadow is thinner than the soft palate shadow (Fig. 13.7), **REFER**.

● In both children and adults, check ears for secretory otitis media, as this may be due to eustachian tube obstruction caused by nasopharyngeal masses.

● Palpate the neck thoroughly in adults to exclude clinically enlarged cervical lymph nodes from a nasopharyngeal carcinoma.

PITFALLS

● Rhinitis medicamentosa arises from prolonged use of non-steroidal topical applications which should, therefore, be avoided. The nasal mucosa swells to cause blockage as a result of these prolonged applications; further dosage, although relieving the blockage temporarily, causes further swelling, etc. If the patient has presented with blockage after self-medication, **REFER** as these cases may require surgical help.

● Unilateral nasal discharge in children is a foreign body until otherwise proven; unless the foreign body is obvious at the nasal vestibule, in which case it can be hooked out. **REFER URGENTLY** .

- Children should not be diagnosed as having polyps except in cystic fibrosis; swollen inferior turbinates are often mistaken for polypi.

- The word 'catarrh' is nebulous and should not be used.

- Immigrant patients from hot climates (with relatively sparse fomites) may take a couple of years to show symptoms of house-dust allergy.

- A unilateral nasal polyp in an adult, with or without bleeding, should be **REFERRED** to exclude an underlying neoplasm.

- For longterm intranasal steroid maintenance treatment, drops should be avoided to prevent significant systemic absorption.

- Be aware of the inspiratory valvular component in nasal blockage.

- If cacosmia and facial pain occur, secondary paranasal sepsis should be suspected and should be **REFERRED** for antral lavage.

14

Epistaxis

Patients usually present with recurrent bleeding, often spontaneous, from one or both nostrils. Epistaxis from trauma may present to the GP but more frequently to an Accident and Emergency
Department.

CHILDREN

Children tend to bleed from varicose vessels over the anterior part
of the septum known as the Little's area; i.e. that which can be
seen when the nasal tip is tilted upwards (Fig. 14.1)

Bleeding may be associated with:

- Coryza
- Exacerbation of allergic rhinitis
- Nose-picking
- Vestibulitis

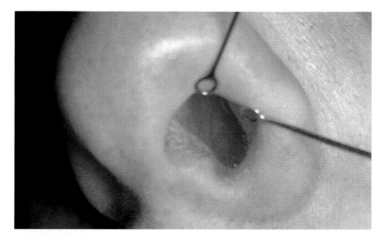

Fig. 14.1 Little's area is that area of the septum seen through the nostrils when the
nasal tip is tilted upwards; anastomic vessels in this area are prone to become
varicose and bleed.

- Foreign body associated with foul discharge
- May be prodromal to exanthematous infections

Management

- Bleeds from Little's area can normally be arrested by pinching the nasal vestibules, i.e. the soft parts of the nasal tip. This should be associated with leaning forward to prevent blood entering the postnasal space.

- Cauterise with silver nitrate sticks after 5 min application of 4% lignocaine on cottonwool (Fig. 14.2). This should be followed by local application of an antibiotic/antiseptic cream for 5–7 days.

- If no vessel is apparent because of slough or crusting over Little's area, apply antibiotic/antiseptic cream for one week, then review.

- If there is no obvious bleeding point, consider blood dyscrasia or diathesis.
- For repeated bleeds **REFER**.

ADULTS

- Anterior bleeds from Little's area: treat as for children (above).

- Posterior bleeds: these are suspected if no bleeding point can be seen anteriorly and cannot be stopped by pinching the nasal vestibules.

- Posterior bleeds:
  - occur more often in later life
  - are more severe in hypertension

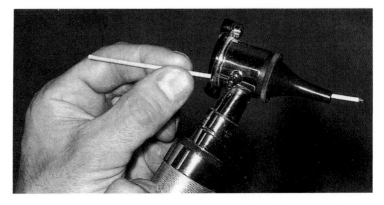

Fig. 14.2 The auriscope with a wide speculum provides magnification and light for chemical cautery to Little's area; the lens is swung to the side to allow access.

- may stop spontaneously
- often present to the Accident and Emergency Department where the nose may be packed and the patient admitted

Management

Anterior bleeds

- Treat with silver nitrate cautery and antibiotic/antiseptic (as for children).

Posterior bleeds

- Check blood pressure.
- If recurrent, **REFER**.
- If an intranasal mass is visible **REFER**.

PITFALLS

- Check to see if the patient is on anticoagulants or aspirin-based drugs.

- Check for signs of thrombocytopaenia and bleeding diatheses: **REFER** to a haematologist.

- In adolescent males, angiofibroma should be considered if substantial nasal blockage is present. **REFER** if no obvious bleeding from the septum.

15

Sinusitis

The diagnosis is frequently suspected in general practice. The following symptoms and signs are suggestive of sinusitis at initial presentation and usually occur after a viral URTI:

- Cacosmia
- Facial + frontal pain and tenderness
- Nasal blockage
- Mucopurulent rhinorrhoea
- Feverishness associated with above

Peri-orbital or frontal swellings (Pott's puffy tumour) may complicate sinusitis when infection is unchecked or inadequately treated; this scenario is unusual nowadays.

Associated constitutional symptoms in sinusitis may be:

- Sensation of congestion in face, head and ears
- Light-headedness

On this basis, it would be reasonable to treat this initial presentation as an **acute rhinosinusitis**.

MANAGEMENT

Acute rhinosinusitis

- If peri-orbital and frontal swellings, **REFER** to ENT department

- The anaerobic environment within the infected sinus calls for use of metronidazole; penicillin or erythromycin should be added to deal with aerobic pathogens

- Give analgesics

- Menthol and steam inhalations reduce the discomfort of nasal blockage

- Should resolution fail **REFER**

Recurrent rhinosinusitis

Pain/aching of the supraorbital ridge(s) behind the eye(s) is frequently diagnosed as recurrent rhinosinusitis. In the absence of any correlated nasal symptoms as described above, other referred causes should be strongly considered, e.g:

- Tension of muscles at the base of skull or neck
- Cervical spondylosis

Both these musculoskeletal conditions become apparent at clinical examination; painful trigger points are easily identifiable and often produce referred pain to that side of the face or head. For these conditions arrange physiotherapy or cervical collar with or without standard musculoskeletal medication.

The diagnosis of **recurrent rhinosinusitis** is therefore established by the symptoms of headache closely associated with nasal symptoms as outlined previously and will serve as a basis for rational management.

The suggested way forward would be along clinical lines to establish whether the patient has a truly infective problem or causes are other than infection such as:

- Allergic rhinitis (see Ch. 13) which would cause mucosal swelling and compromise ethmoidal, antral and frontal ventilation

- Unilateral or bilateral middle turbinate impaction of the septum producing referred symptoms of facial or temporal pain (see Fig 15.1): **REFER**

- Polypi which may be noticed arising from the middle meati; in conjunction with the symptoms these should be treated as given in Chapter 13

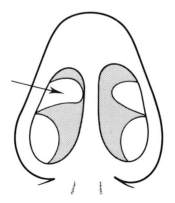

Fig. 15.1 Middle turbinate impaction on the septum.

Imaging

Although sinus X-rays have been the traditional approach towards diagnosis, any finding other than fluid levels (Fig. 15.2) is unhelpful and probably renders the investigation unnecessary.

With recurrent or refractory cases the ENT–orientated GP may wish to request a CT scan series of sinuses (high resolution coronal); this is now a cost-effective and accessible investigation to identify any predisposing bony anomalies and show the extent of mucosal disease.

Typical bony anomalies which may appear on the radiologist's report would include:

- Concha bullosa (a middle turbinate expanded by an air cell) (Fig. 15.3)

- Paradoxically bent middle turbinate.

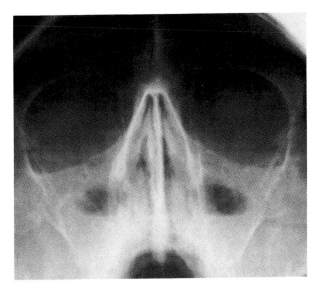

Figure 15.2 Occipo-mental view of maxillary antra to assess fluid level.

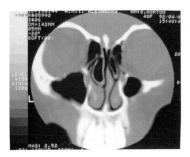

Fig. 15.3 CT scan of sinuses showing concha bullosa.

A CT scan free of any mucosal swelling or impaction of bony anomalies would itself be helpful in excluding paranasal and sinus disease.

Treatment

(1) Cases whom the GP can help

- Acute exacerbations of a recurrent infective picture which require the use of:
  - Metronidazole to cover likely anaerobes as well as erythromycin or penicillin
  - Analgesics
  - Menthol and steam inhalations to reduce discomfort or nasal blockage

- Allergic rhinitis (see Ch. 13). Intranasal steroid sprays are often useful. If steroid sprays fail because of poor nasal patency, such patients need $\boxed{REFERRAL}$ for inferior turbinate shrinkage. Intranasal steroids are contraindicated where there is radiographic evidence of paranasal sepsis; $\boxed{REFER}$ for diagnostic washout.

- Small nasal polypi may respond to intranasal sprays or intranasal steroid drops; if pus is seen, cover with antibiotics (as above).

(2) Cases requiring $\boxed{REFERRAL}$

- Recurrent infections should be $\boxed{REFERRED}$ for further assessment and possible surgery on the lateral nasal wall using modern endoscopic equipment
- Adverse CT result
- Large nasal polypi for excision
- Gross septal deviations
- Suspected antro-ethmoidal carcinoma

PITFALLS

- Postnasal drip alone is a non-specific symptom and is often environmentally related.

- In uncomplicated sinusitis, facial swelling does not occur. Facial swelling tenderness indicates dental abscess, $\boxed{REFER}$ to dental practitioner.

- Facial expansion with ipselateral blood-stained nasal discharge may represent a neoplasm; check for proptosis, cheimosis, palatal expansion and diminished hemipalatal sensation on that side.

- Perorbital cellulitis presenting (in children especially) implies that sinusitis has progressed into the anterior peri-orbital tissue via the ethmoid cells. **REFER** for parenteral antibiotic treatment as an in-patient.

- Frontal swellings in relation to a suspected diagnosis of sinustitis should be **REFERRED** to exclude frontal osteo-myelitis, mucocele or large osteoma.

- Rhinitis medicamentosa can be avoided by restricting intra-nasal medications to steroidal types.

16

Sore throat

This is one of the commonest presenting symptoms in general practice and will occupy a great deal of thought if the most appropriate management plan is to be chosen.

In reality patients describe an array of symptoms that fall within a spectrum ranging from mild to severe and characterised by:

Mild viral pharyngitis

- Sore or dry throat
- Worse in morning
- No constitutional disturbance
- Patient may be aware of nasal obstruction, especially at night
- Associated coryza

Bacterial tonsillitis (which can be severe)

- Sore throat
- Severe malaise
- Pyrexia
- Cervical lymphadenopathy
- Referred earache
- Halitosis

THE GP'S APPROACH TO THE SORE THROAT

- The initial approach is to elicit the features as listed above by a detailed history.

- Inspection of GP records will give clues as to the duration and frequency of previous episodes.

- Examination will reveal a spectrum of abnormalities depending on severity.

With a viral aetiology, the signs may be

- Minimal generalised pharyngeal vascular injection
- Ulceration of faucial arches and soft palate which, if unilateral, may indicate herpes zoster (Ramsay-Hunt)
- Palatal petechiae
- Uvular oedema
- Cold sores (herpes simplex I) on lips or nostrils

With bacterial aetiology, acute signs may be

- Aggressive injection and swelling limited to the tonsils and faucial pillars
- Crypts full of pus suggestive, but not diagnostic, of tonsillitis; crypts can contain pus even when quiescent
- Fetor
- Plummy speech
- Facial flushing
- Pyrexia
- Tender cervical lymphadenopathy
- General malaise

Glandular fever (syn. infectious mononucleosis)

This severe Epstein-Barr viral illness is characterised by

- Fetor
- Plummy speech
- Slough on grossly swollen tonsils (Fig.16.1)
- Palatal petechiae

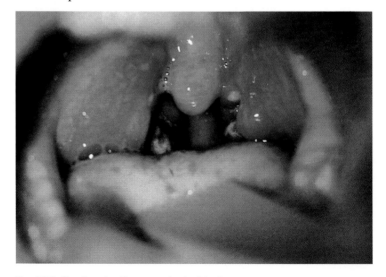

Fig. 16.1 Slough on tonsils as seen in glandular fever.

- Pyrexia
- LKKS and general lymphadenopathy
- General malaise

MANAGEMENT OF SORE THROAT

The patient or parent of a young patient invariably has preconceived ideas, concerns and expectations. It is likely they perceive that any episode of sore throat represents bacterial tonsillitis for which they expect to receive antibiotics; this misconception may well be based on previous treatment patterns.

- The patient will benefit from aspirin gargles (600 mg 4 times a day) but not in children, asthmatics or dyspeptics. This drug works topically on inflamed mucosa and need not be swallowed.

- Paracetamol is useful as an antipyretic and systemic analgesic.

- The majority of patients with sore throats have probably managed themselves for a day or so with simple analgesics before presenting themselves at the GP's surgery.

At this stage, it has to be decided whether an antibiotic is going to be beneficial; this is a genuinely difficult decision if treatment is to be optimal, both clinically and economically. The elements of the history as previously outlined, in conjunction with severe constitutional disturbance, will call for antibiotics, e.g. phenoxymethylpenicillin or erythromycin for 10 days. This duration of treatment is suggested as the relapse rate has been shown to be lower than with the 5–7 day regimes.

Ampicillin-based drugs should be avoided if glandular fever is initially suspected or whilst awaiting a *monospot* result.

The patient may actually present with or progress to a complication of bacterial tonsillitis in the form of:

Peritonsillar cellulitis

This is the presuppurative stage of quinsy and always develops from tonsillitis and will also show:

- Unilateral peritonsillar swelling and redness
- Relatively little trismus (spasm of pterygoid muscles preventing opening of the mouth)

Quinsy

This is the next stage and represents a localised collection of pus above the tonsil. The features are:

- Those of peritonsillar cellulitis
- Trismus

Both these conditions are severely debilitating and require in-patient treatment in the form of drainage (if applicable), intravenous access for hydration and antibiotic. $\boxed{\textbf{\textit{REFER}}}$ for admission.

CONSIDERATION FOR TONSILLECTOMY

There are two main indications for tonsillectomy: recurrent infection and mechanical blockage in its own right or a combination of both. It is helpful to consider the following points:

- Traditional dogma of frequency and age is too simplistic to be helpful.
- The decision is multifactorial taking into account:
  - Frequency and severity
  - Parental reaction to the child's illness
  - General failure to thrive
  - Occasional cases of chronic low-grade pharyngitis between attacks.
- It would be useful to explore the thoughts of your ENT consultant colleagues.
- Sometimes the tonsils can be so hypertrophied as to obstruct breathing and swallowing; tonsillectomy for these problems is immensely beneficial.

MANAGEMENT OF RECURRENT OR CHRONIC PHARYNGITIS

- Check nasal patency; chronic mouth-breathing will dry and irritate the throat (see Ch. 13).
- Discourage smoking and chronic use of proprietary throat lozenges or sprays.
- If the pharyngitis is secondary to nasal obstruction and has not responded to oral decongestants or intranasal steroids $\boxed{\textbf{\textit{REFER}}}$.

MANAGEMENT OF GLANDULAR FEVER

- *Monospot* and film are advised to confirm a clinical diagnosis about a fortnight after onset.
- 20% of negative *monospot* results convert to positive during the course of the illness.
- Constitutional disturbance invariably occurs and should be managed appropriately.
- Prolonged periods of rest will be required and the condition may take months to settle, waxing and waning as it does so; this should be explained to the patient.

- Subtle changes in liver function tests are common but clinically overt liver dysfunction is rare. It is worth advising a low-fat diet in the early phase.
- Additional depression may require separate treatment.

OTHER CAUSES OF PHARYNGITIS

- Iatrogenic from prolonged antibiotics for other disorders resulting in candidal pharyngitis (Fig. 16.2)
- NSAID usage causing agranulocytosis
- Gross dental caries; requires dental REFERRAL
- Tobacco
- Gastro-oesophageal reflux of acid/bile
- Alcohol overuse
- Occupational irritants
- Voice abuse: consider speech therapy REFERRAL
- Styloid pain is elicited by palpating the tonsil on the affected side with a gloved finger: REFER
- Venereal infection

PITFALLS

- Unilaterally sore or enlarged tonsil, in the absence of acute inflammation, is strongly suggestive of neoplasia: REFER.

- Ampicillin-based drugs as first-line treatment should not be used in suspected glandular fever because a rash can be induced ('poor man's monospot'!).

- Recurrent generalised pharyngitis with worsening debility should prompt a blood film to exclude leukaemia.

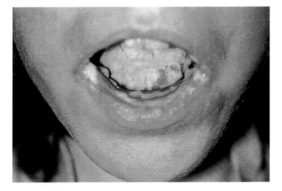

Fig. 16.2 An extreme example of oral candidiasis. This tongue is infected with Candida, which can extend to the pharynx.

17
Hoarseness

This is an abnormality of the voice affecting:

- Pitch
- Volume
- Resonance
- Quality

Hoarseness is often associated with an URTI in the otherwise healthy patient; these are mostly of viral origin.

MANAGEMENT

- Limit the use of the voice to quiet conversation.

- Give analgesic if associated with sore throat.

- Inhale steam from a mixture of hot water and benzoin tincture (5 ml in one pint of hot water).

- Patients with hoarseness that fails to resolve in 2 weeks should be **REFERRED** to exclude neoplasia, nodules or vocal polypi.

FURTHER POINTS OF HISTORY

- Weight-loss suggestive of upper or lower respiratory tract cancer: **REFER**

- Weight-gain suggestive of myxoedema: investigate and treat. **REFER** if hoarseness persists

- Associated dysphagia: suggestive of upper respiratory cancer and palsies of the larynx or pharynx. **REFER**

- Referred earache: possibly an associated symptom of an underlying respiratory tract neoplasm

- Neck swellings: suggest cervical lymphadenopathy, possibly associated with underlying neoplasia

- Contributory suppurative disease
  - sinusitis
  - bronchitis
  - bronchiectasis

- Dyspepsia and gastro-oesophageal reflux

- Chemical trauma
  - industrial
  - smoking

- Voice abuse: can result in the use of the false vocal cords or nodules on the true cords

MANAGEMENT

This is dependent on the treatment of the causative illness, occupation or habit. ENT **REFERRAL** is often mandatory for exclusion of malignancy.

18

Dysphagia

This is difficulty in swallowing (aphagia means inability to swallow) either fluids, solids or both.

POINTS OF HISTORY

Acute

Cases with constitutional disturbance are usually inflammatory:

- Supraglottitis (formerly known as epiglottitis): must be **REFERRED** urgently
- Tonsillitis causing pain, obstruction or both (see Ch. 16)
- Quinsy: **REFER**
- Glandular fever: may need **REFERRAL** for intravenous hydration and steroids if severe

Foreign bodies tend to present to the Accident and Emergency Department but if suspected, **REFER URGENTLY**.

Progressive

Cases which should arouse suspicion of **pharyngeal** or **oesophageal neoplasia** are:

- History of weight-loss and fatigue
- Usually progressively worsening dysphagia for solids to semi-solids to liquids in that order
- Hoarseness
- Cough on drinking suggests aspiration

History suggestive of a benign cause of progressive dysphagia

- Regurgitation of recognisable food suggests a pharyngeal pouch (Fig.18.1). Do a barium swallow to confirm and **REFER**.
- Longstanding acid reflux suggests peptic stricture at the lower end of the oesphagus. **REFER** to surgical or medical colleague.

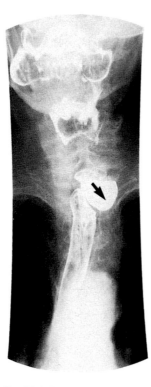

Fig. 18.1 Pharyngeal pouch seen on a barium swallow.

Other problems

- Neurogenic dysphagia may be associated with nasal escape because of palatal paresis along with other cranial nerve palsies. This situation suggests a neoplasm (either primary or secondary) at the base of the skull or a specific neurological condition, e.g. bulbar palsy.

- Connective tissue disorder, e.g. systemic sclerosis.

Prolonged and variable 'lump in throat'

Without constitutional disturbance, this is suggestive of **globus pharyngeus** (formerly known as globus hystericus); the term **pseudodysphagia** is the most satisfactory. This symptom presents a difficult diagnostic problem:

- History of a 'lump in throat' which tends to be relieved by act of swallowing, only to return soon after

- The 'lump' is variable

- No constitutional disturbance

- Possibly an anxiety element because the patient fears the diagnosis of cancer; a relative, friend or neighbour may have had such a diagnosis.

These patients should be ⎡**REFERRED**⎤ for clinical and endoscopic examination which will exclude underlying pathology. It is likely the patient will be referred back to the GP for further general management.

POINTS TO EXCLUDE

On general examination

- Pallid complexion
- Evidence of weight-loss
- Abdominal masses
- Chest findings suggesting secondary infections or consolidations associated with aspiration and chest neoplasm
- Cranial and peripheral nervous system if applicable

On local examination

- Angular cheilitis
- Glossitis
- Neck masses
- Oral masses
  - mouth
  - retromolar trigone (see Glossary)
  - oropharynx (the rest of the pharynx will be examined in the ENT department)
- Movements of
  - tongue
  - palate
  - pharynx
- Sensory examination of the palate and pharynx

MANAGEMENT

Investigations should include:

- Lateral soft tissue X-ray of neck
- Chest X-ray
- Barium swallow
- Full blood count and ESR

If neoplasia or neurogenic cause is suspected, ⎡**REFER**⎤ with the appropriate information.

19

Foreign bodies and local injuries

A GP may encounter these problems in routine practice and the patient can benefit from treatment at primary level locally.

EAR

- Blunt pinna injuries acquired, for example, through contact sports can cause a subperichondrial haematoma (haematoma auris: Fig. 19.1). This requires surgical drainage which is best achieved by an excision of an overlying eliptical piece of skin and perichondrium which prevents premature skin closure. A pressure dressing should be applied and changed daily. A needle drainage is not sufficient as a recollection will occur. The

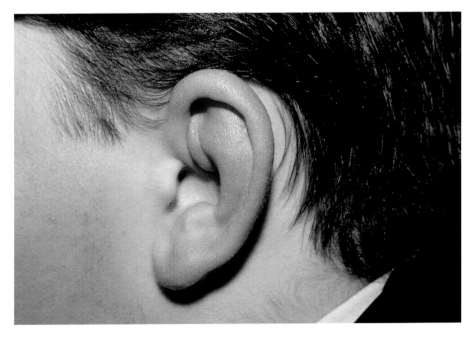

Fig. 19.1 Haematoma auris.

individual practitioner may otherwise ⟨ **REFER** ⟩ the patient to the ENT department urgently; a delay over a few days would result in cartilage necrosis and deformity (cauliflower ear).

- Probing injuries to the meatus and canal are commonly seen in general practice. This is often caused by over-zealous bathroom habits in the use of cotton buds and screwed-up towel corners. On examination there may be seen:
  - A spiral laceration/abrasion of the canal wall, usually posteriorly
  - Traumatic tympanic membrane rupture

  These injuries usually heal spontaneously and do not require active management initially.

- Barotrauma to the tympanic membrane is caused by a pressure wave from a slap or similar force; a blast from an explosion would cause similar damage. The tympanic perforation is usually situated posteriorly and should heal spontaneously in 6 weeks. Pressure changes during aircraft flight descent can very occasionally cause this damage but usually with a co-existent otitis media.

- Foreign bodies in the ear can stretch the most fertile imagination; insects should be swamped with olive oil and other items such as small beads and bits of cotton wool should be syringed gently.

NOSE

- Nasal injuries can result in damage to skin, bone, cartilage or a combination of these.

- Isolated skin lacerations can be closed by sutures or self-adhesive strips.

- Bony damage can merely be bruising of the periostium and overlying skin and it is prudent therefore to allow the skin swelling and bruising to settle over 7–10 days before a judgement can be made about whether there is an underlying displaced fracture. Simple analgesia may be used meanwhile. If a new deviation has occurred, then a manipulation may return the bony bridge to its original shape. Should the patient wish to take this option, ⟨ **REFER** ⟩ to the local ENT department for manipulation within 3 weeks at most from the date of injury as bone unition is well under way by then.

  If there is no deviation after 7–10 days but yet the nose is tender, this very likely represents an undisplaced fracture which merely requires analgesia.

- X-rays do not contribute to the clinical management but would

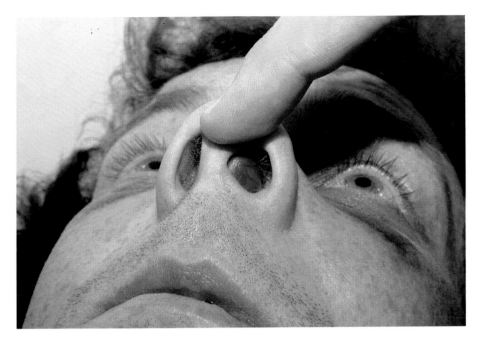

Fig. 19.2 Septal haematoma.

be expected from the medico-legal point of view with regard to personal injury claims.

● Cartilage injuries usually affect the septum and fall into two categories: septal haematoma (Fig. 19.2) and deviations. Septal haematoma presents with a soft bulging of the septum on one or both sides; **REFER** for drainage to prevent subsequent tip collapse.

● Foreign bodies present with a foul unilateral blood-stained discharge and usually require **REFERRAL** to an ENT department for removal.

THROAT

● The usual presentation in general practice is a non-acute sensation of a foreign body stuck in the throat. Small items, e.g. fish bones, can occasionally be seen lodged in the tonsil and removed with forceps. Most patients will require **REFERRAL** to an ENT department for further examination.

20

The primary health care team

Most GPs are part of a team of health care workers. These people can help in the handling of ENT problems in the community and comprise:

THE PRACTICE NURSE

This member of the team can be trained by the local ENT department for the following tasks:

- Perform ear syringing

- Introduce ½ inch ribbon gauze wicks into ears

- Arrest nose bleeds by squeezing the tip of the nose over the Little's area (Fig. 20.1)

- Perform audiograms if the practice has access to audiometry equipment

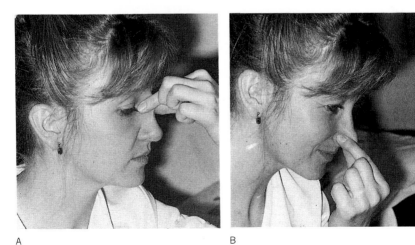

A   B

Fig. 20.1 A Pinching the bones will not stop a nosebleed. **B** Pinching the nasal vestibules onto the anterior septum will compress culpable vessels in Little's area.

- Arrange a local mastoid cavity cleaning clinic if needed
- Take venous blood samples and swabs where appropriate

THE HEALTH VISITOR

- Often the primary contact with parents who suspect a hearing problem in their baby
- Performs routine hearing tests

  0–6 months: 'startle' reflex
  6–9 months: distraction test
  16–30 months: cooperative test
  3–5 years: toy discrimination test and pure-tone sweep frequency test

- Assesses speech and language development
- Arranges pure-tone audiometry for children at the local audiometry department

THE DISTRICT NURSE

- Performs ear syringing at a patient's home
- Assists with giving medicine at a patient's home
- Performs tracheostomy care (Fig. 20.2)
- Liaises with the palliative care nurse in some cases of malignancy

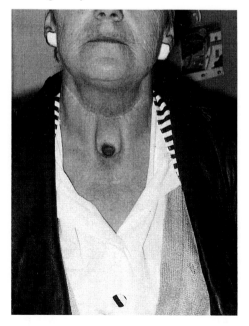

Fig. 20.2 This tracheostomy is part of a total laryngectomy.

THE SCHOOL MEDICAL OFFICER

- Performs primary and secondary school entry hearing tests and receives support from school nurses, educational psychologists and speech therapists

- May well refer cases of suspected deafness to a ENT clinic whence correspondence will be sent to the GP

PRIVATE HEARING CENTRES

- Some patients may self-refer to these services. The centre may send a report of their findings and actions to the GP.

21

GP and ENT postoperative sequelae

Most treatments concerning ENT postoperative care will be conducted by the ENT department. However the following are some ENT problems which, more often than not, present to the GP rather than the hospital department:

POST-TONSILLECTOMY BLEEDING

Reactive bleeding

This takes place **within 48 hours of tonsillectomy** and is due either to a ligature slipping or a vessel opening spontaneously. As the patient is very likely to be in hospital at the time of this particular emergency, it is unlikely to be seen at home. **Emergency re-admission to hospital** is clearly necessary.

Secondary bleeding

This occurs within 5–10 days of the operation and the patient is likely to be at home. The traditional teaching is that secondary bleeding occurs as a result of an infection in the tonsillar fossae but there is little evidence to support this. More likely it is due to a piece of granulation tissue having separated. The patient should be **REFERRED URGENTLY** to the ENT department where admission will be arranged for a day or two for careful observation with or without antibiotic treatment depending on the policy of the particular surgeon. Secondary bleeding is usually less brisk than reactive bleeds.

Postoperative pain

Although the patient is usually released from hospital with suitable oral analgesia, postoperative throat pain, including referred earache, often gets worse 3 days or so postoperatively once the patient is at home (Fig. 21.1). The GP is sometimes called at this

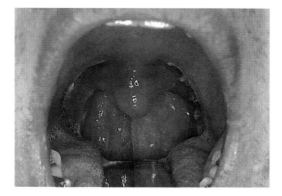

Fig. 21.1 Postoperative slough in the tonsillar fossae.

point; a common error is to misconstrue normal proteinaceous exudate for pus and infection.

- If post-operative antibiotics were started postoperatively by the ENT department as a matter of policy, this drug will be substituted for another in the mistaken belief of an infection. The patient is usually apyrexial and will respond well to the addition of **diclofenac** although this is contraindicated in asthma.

- For children use **paracetamol mucilage** or **ibuprofen elixir** (although contraindicated in asthma).

- The cause of the late pain reaction is the leisurely deposition of post-traumatic inflammatory substances.

- In the unlikely event of a pyrexia, infection should be clearly considered.

- Although **earache** is usually referred, the tympanic membranes should nevertheless be examined to exclude otitis media. Temporomandibular joint pain is most unusual in this context.

General points

- In the midst of distress, the adult patient or the parent of a young patient may regret the whole business of having submitted to the operation. Careful explanation is required and encouragement that, after 2 weeks, everything will have settled.

- As far as food is concerned, rough textures such as nuts, crisps and fruit, eaten little and often will keep the throat clean and the underlying muscles active; battling with one or two large meals a day should be discouraged, as should languishing exclusively with ice-creams and jellies.

ADENOIDECTOMY

- **Postoperative bleeding** into the mouth should prompt **urgent readmission** with a view to postnasal packing.

- **Postoperative pain** after adenoidectomy is minimal, if any. Referred earache should not be diagnosed until the tympanic membranes have been examined to exclude otitis media.

GROMMETS

The GP will sometimes be consulted about a **discharge** from an ear which has recently had a grommet (Fig. 21.2) inserted. This may occur as a result of an URTI or contamination, such as swimming-bath water.

Management

- A 5-day course of antibiotic ear drops properly applied (see Ch. 4) should clear this or at least improve matters.

- Should this fail, the patient should be sent to the ENT department for further evaluation with a view to grommet removal.

- Parents will nearly all ask whether their child can **swim with grommets**. There is now evidence to show that children with grommets who swim do not have any more trouble that those who have been forbidden. Advice will still vary from surgeon to surgeon but sensible advice would be to advocate some form of ear plug and avoidance of ducking and diving; this topic will usually be covered by the staff of the ENT department.

- Shampoos and conditioners in the ears should also be avoided.

NASAL SURGERY

Pain is unusual postoperatively. Nasal splints, sometimes inserted to prevent the formation of adhesions, may occasionally cause distressing pain; this is due to the pressure of the splints or the suture used to secure the splints.

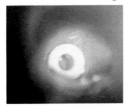

Fig. 21.2 This grommet is ventilating the middle ear via the lumen through which the middle ear mucosa can be seen. the colour of the grommet material will vary according to the manufacturer.

- If there are no obvious signs of infection, analgesics will help.

- If there is swelling or gross infection of the nasal tip the patient should be $\boxed{\textbf{\textit{REFERRED}}}$ back to the ENT department.

Epistaxis

Epistaxis should be redirected to the ENT department. Blood staining of mucous discharge is usually a reaction to surgical trauma and will soon settle.

- The use of cotton wool rather than paper tissue to wipe the nose will help prevent a frictional vestibulitis of the nose.

- An **antibiotic cream** is a useful adjunct and should be applied twice a day for 5 days.

22

Glossary of specialist vocabulary commonly used in correspondence from ENT departments

This list is clearly not comprehensive of all the specialist terms, some of which will be used within the realms of other specialities and will therefore be more widely known.

Acoustic neuroma: A schwannoma of the vestibular division of the auditory nerve; this is benign although pressure symptoms render it life-threatening if the tumour is large.

Anosmia: Lack of sense of smell.

Antrostomy: A commonly used term for intranasal antrostomy which is the creation of a large hole in the inferior meatus between the nasal cavity and the ipselateral maxillary sinus. This is being superseded by functional endoscopic sinus surgery where the antrostomy is placed in the middle meatus to which the antral ciliary flow function is naturally directed.

Audiogram: A *pure-tone audiogram* is a chart of the pure-tone thresholds at various frequencies. A *speech audiogram* is a graph illustrating the ability of the subject to discriminate between similarly sounding words and may be used in conjunction with other tests to differentiate between cochlear and auditory nerve deafness.

Brain stem evoked response: A measure of auditory pathway electrical activity in response to clicking sounds. This is an objective test, over which the patient has no control, as opposed to pure-tone and speech audiometry where the patient's subjective response is recorded.

Cacosmia: A subjective unpleasant smell.

Cageusia: A bad taste in the mouth.

Caldwell-Luc: A surgical approach to the maxillary antrum via an incision above the upper canine and premolar teeth. Once the antrum is entered, irreversibly inflamed mucosa can be stripped away. An intranasal antrostomy is usually done at the same time to allow easy access to wash out postoperative blood clots and debris. This operation is usually reserved for end-stage mucosal disease.

Caloric test: The assessment of labyrinthine function by warm or cold fluid application to the tympanic membrane; in cases of tympanic perforation, cold and warm air is used. The duration of the resulting nystagmus is recorded and compared one side with the other. A conclusion can, therefore, be drawn as to whether a particular labyrinth is paretic.

Choanal atresia: A congenital absence of a posterior nasal passageway; this can be either unilateral or bilateral.

Cholesteatoma: An encysted collection of squamous epithelial debris, usually originating in the upper reaches of the middle ear and often involving the mastoid antrum. It has erosive properties by virtue of osteolytic enzymes and bony Haversian canal plugging.

Cricopharyngeal myotomy: Surgical splitting of the cricopharyngeus muscle at the top of the oesophagus, performed either internally or externally to assist in the management of a **pharyngeal pouch**. When performed internally through an endoscope, it is often referred to as Dohlman's operation. The more recent technique of endoscopic stapling and division of the cricopharyngeal bar has been gaining favour.

Cricothyrotomy: A surgically produced hole in the cricothyroid membrane as an alternative to a tracheostomy, in order to relieve upper respiratory obstruction.

Dohlman's operation: An endoscopic approach to performing cricopharyngeal myotomy using diathermy (cf. cricopharyngeal myotomy).

Dysarthria: Incoordinate enunciation of speech.

Dysphasia: A disorder of symbolic function of speech, distorting understanding and verbal expression.

Dysphonia: Abnormality of pitch, volume, resonance or quality of voice.

Electrocochleogram: An objective measurement of electrical activity of the cochlea in response to clicking sounds. In children, this usually requires a short general anaesthetic.

Epiglottitis: A clinical emergency arising from an acute inflammation and oedema of the epiglottis and surrounding supraglottic tissues; the term **supraglottitis** is now more commonly used.

Ethmoiditis: Inflammation of the ethmoid cells, thought to be contributory to the formation of nasal polyps.

Functional endoscopic sinus surgery: The use of rigid fibre-optic telescopes is taking on increasing importance; the concept is to restore sinus ventilation and ciliary flow of mucus with minimum disruption to the lateral nasal wall; this approach is not only more physiological but less traumatic than the older 'blunderbuss' treatments.

Furuncle: A boil of hair follicle in the skin of the outer third of the external auditory meatus; the inner two-thirds of the canal skin does not contain hair follicles.

Globus syndrome: A sensation of a lump in the throat *without* true dysphagia. The term globus hystericus is incorrect and has been superseded by two terms: **globus pharyngeus** and **pseudodysphagia**.

Glomus tumour: A tumour of baroreceptor tissue in (a) internal jugular vein, (b) middle ear, (c) the vagus nerve as it emerges from the skull.

Glossitis: Inflammation of the tongue.

Glossodynia: painful tongue; this symptom may not have any demonstrable physical basis.

Glottis: Synonymous with the true vocal cords. The area above is called the **supraglottis** and the area below the **subglottis**.

Glue ear: A term often used for an effusion in the middle ear whose synonyms are serious otitis media, otitis media with effusion, secretory otitis media and catarrhal otitis.

Grommet: A tiny tube which is inserted into the tympanic membrane to improve middle ear ventilation; these tubes are made in a variety of materials and designs. They usually (but not always) migrate from the tympanic membrane within 3–12 months of insertion unless specifically designed for permanent retention.

Herpes zoster oticus: A herpes zoster infection of the geniculate ganglion in the temporal bone causing ipselateral lower motor neurone facial palsy and painful rash of the external ear, palate, pharynx and rarely the larynx. There may be associated sensorineural deafness; the term **Ramsay-Hunt syndrome** is used synonymously.

Incudostapedial joint: The joint of articulation between the long process of incus and the head of the stapes. It can be disrupted by chronic retraction of the tympanic membrane over the joint, chronic suppurative otitis media, recurrent acute otitis media and severe trauma, either accidental or surgical.

Inverted papilloma: Otherwise known as **transitional cell papilloma**, arising from nasal or sinus mucosa. Rarely premalignant.

Keratosis obturans: An accumulation of debris in the deep part of the external auditory canal causing painful erosion of the surrounding bone; thought to be due to defective epithelial migration along the external auditory canal.

Laryngocele: An abnormal herniation of the laryngeal mucosa between true and false cords. This may well present with a lump in the neck, worsened by blowing against a resistance, e.g. trumpets. Swelling can appear externally, internally (in the valleculae) or both.

Laryngectomy: Removal of larynx either partially or totally. Depending on the amount of thyroid tissue removed, thyroid and parathyroid hormone replacement may be required.

Laryngomalacia: Synonymously known as a floppy larynx which is a self-curing infantile condition presenting with stridor.

Lermoyez syndrome: A variant of Ménière's syndrome, where tinnitus and deafness are relieved by the onset of vertigo.

Leukoplakia: Literally, a white patch caused by dysplastic or early malignant squamous epithelium.

Ludwig's angina: Cellulitis of the floor of the mouth and neck, caused by haemolytic streptococcus.

Mastoidectomy: An operation to remove diseased mastoid bone. A *radical mastoidectomy* is performed in the management of cholesteatoma. A *modified radical mastoidectomy* is a radical mastoidectomy with preservation or reconstruction of parts of the ossicles and tympanic membrane. A *corticol mastoidectomy* is performed for mucosal disease and is less commonly used than formerly.

Ménière's syndrome: A quartet of symptoms: prodromal sensation of fullness in the ear, along with vertigo which is associated with variable hearing and tinnitus. The syndrome is the clinical manifestation of Ménière's disease which encompasses the syndrome with the known microscopic abnormalities of the cochlea.

Microcordotomy: A linear incision (under microscopic control) along the upper surface of the true vocal cords to release chronic Reinke's oedema. This procedure preserves the integrity of the vocal cord epithelium and mucosal wave.

Mucosal wave: This refers to the rippling of the vocal cord epithelium during phonation; the pattern starts from the underside and progresses towards the upper surface. This wave can be studied during stroboscopic laryngoscopy.

Myringitis: Inflammation, usually granular or bullous, specifically of the tympanic membrane.

Myringostome: A less commonly used synonym for a tympanic membrane perforation.

Myringotomy: A small incision made in the tympanic membrane to release middle ear fluid; this incisional site allows insertion of a grommet.

Nystagmus: Involuntary oscillation of the eyes, having two components: slow and fast. The slow phase is due to the labyrinth disorder itself and the fast phase is due to cortical correction. By convention, it is the direction of the fast phase which is used to label the direction of nystagmus.

Olser's syndrome: A foreshortened term which should really include the names of Weber and Rendu, synonymous with hereditary telangectasia and often presenting with epistaxis.

Otorrhagia: Specifically bleeding from the ear.

Otorrhoea: The general term for discharge from the ear; this word should be qualified by the type of discharge, e.g. mucous.

Otosclerosis: A proliferation of bone derived from the otic capsule; in practical terms, otosclerosis applies to an area of proliferation of bone around the stapes footplate.

Ozaena: An unpleasant smell emanting from the nose due to atrophic rhinitis. The smell is noticed by those around although uncommonly by the sufferer because of the damage to the olfactory epithelium.

Pharyngeal pouch: Synonymous with hypopharyngeal pouch and Zenker's diverticulum. An abnormal herniation of mucosa between a thyropharyngeus and a cricopharyngeus in the lower reaches of the pharynx.

Pharyngo-laryngectomy: Removal of both larynx and pharynx, the latter being reconstructed by various techniques of grafting, e.g. free jejunal. Thyroid and parathyroid hormone replacement is invariably necessary.

Polyp: A macroscopic term regardless of histology to describe a pedunculated mass, not necessarily neoplastic, attached to a surface. A nasal polyp really represents swollen and pedunculated mucosa from the lateral nasal wall; an aural polyp represents granulation tissue although presenting macroscopically in a polypoid shape.

Presbycusis: The wear and tear of the cochlear hair cells.

Quinsy: An abscess (localised collection of pus) above the tonsil.

Rannula: A mucosal cystic swelling in the floor of the mouth.

Reinke's oedema: Swelling of both vocal cords due to subepithelial oedema.

Retromolar trigone: Area in the mouth between the lower back teeth and side of tongue; exposed clinically by retracting the tongue away from the teeth. This should be carefully examined in a case of an unexplained neck lump.

Rhinorrhoea: A nasal discharge; the term should be qualified by the quality of discharge, e.g. watery.

Sialadenitis: Inflammation of the salivary glands.

Speech valve: This is inserted either at the time of laryngectomy or at a later stage in order to restore speech. There is a wide range of longevity for these valves and they can be replaced as required. The speech and language therapists are closely involved with the assessment and routine management.

Stridor: Abnormal laryngeal sounds, specific to the respiratory cycle.

Stapedectomy: An operation to relieve the conductive deafness of **otosclerosis**. The stapes and some or all of the footplate is removed and replaced with a prosthesis. This operation is not without its risks and therefore not always an appropriate primary option; a hearing aid may be considered first.

Supraglottis: The area of the larynx above the glottis or true vocal cords.

Subglottis: The area of the larynx below the glottis or true vocal cords.

Tracheostomy: A surgically fashioned hole from the exterior into the trachea to relieve upper respiratory obstruction.

Tracheotomy: The surgical action of making the hole in the trachea.

Tympanoplasty: Surgical repair of middle ear sound conduction mechanism. In effect, a tympanoplasty is a myringoplasty with surgical attention to the ossicles as well.

Tympanosclerosis: Chalk patches deposited within the substance of the tympanic membrane as a result of inflammation which has organised. These chalk patches can also occur in the mucosa around the ossicles.

Tympanotomy: An incision in the posterior meatal wall to lift up the external auditory canal skin in continuity with the tympanic membrane so that the middle ear can be exposed for diagnostic inspection or surgical procedures. The incision is used, for example, in stapedectomy, where a plastic prosthesis is inserted in place of a fixed stapes bone.

UVPPP: This stands for uvulo-palato-pharyngoplasty which is one of the operations to deal with severe snoring.

Vertigo: A hallucination of rotary movement; not to be confused with light-headedness.

Index